This Is A Comma In Your Life, Not A Period

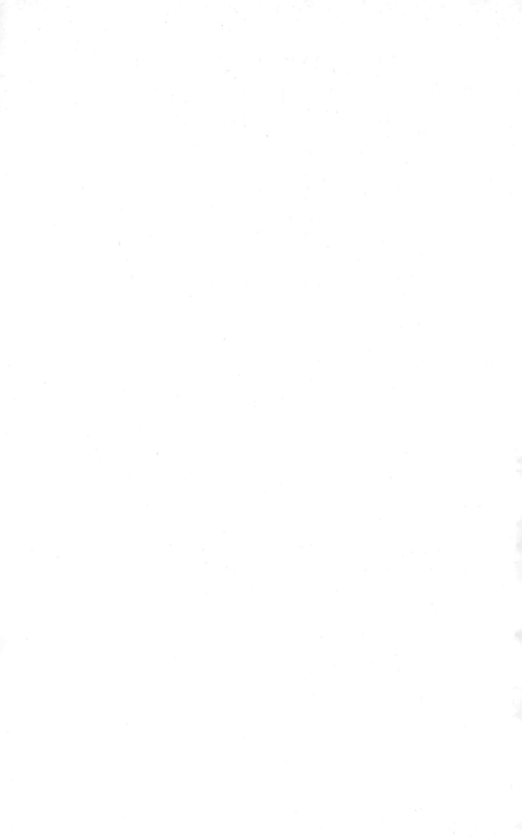

This Is A Comma In Your Life, Not A Period

Finishing Strong On Your Journey To Emotional, Physical, And Spiritual Healing

Dr. Tunishai A. Ford

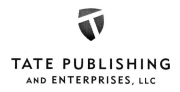

TATE PUBLISHING
AND ENTERPRISES, LLC

Published by Tate Publishing & Enterprises, LLC
127 E. Trade Center Terrace | Mustang, Oklahoma 73064 USA
1.888.361.9473 | www.tatepublishing.com

Tate Publishing is committed to excellence in the publishing industry. The company reflects the philosophy established by the founders, based on Psalm 68:11,
"The Lord gave the word and great was the company of those who published it."

Book design copyright © 2014 by Tate Publishing, LLC. All rights reserved.

Published in the United States of America

ISBN: 978-1-63122-381-5
1. Health & Fitness / Diseases / Cancer
2. Body, Mind & Spirit / Inspiration & Personal Growth
13.12.26

Contents

1. The Moment Of Truth   1

2. The Prognosis And Treatment   21

3. A Rude Awakening   41

4. God Hears A Mother's Prayer   73

5. An Angel Named Tee   85

6. Vernetta's Song   91

7. The Inner Healing   99

8. The Victory   113

9. This Is A Comma In Your Life, Not A Period   123

10. Conclusion: Finishing Strong   135

Super Antioxidant Tonic   145

Poem: What Cancer Cannot Do   148

Poem: This is a Comma in Your Life, Not a Period

       149

Book Highlights From This Is A Comma In Your Life, Not A Period   151

Dedication

To my precious mother, Corliss Ford,
who departed this life on April 4, 2006.

Your loving words and encouragement
will always drive me to strive
and live the abundant life that you
so desired for me and all your other children.

Now, you are embracing God
and is forever glowing in his presence.

I love you forever.

Acknowledgments

I first give thanks to my Lord and Savior, Jesus Christ, who healed me from the inside out and allowed me to write this book to be a blessing to others.

To my sister, Rev. Marlene Gingrich-Milarski, for the many prayers and encouragement you gave me. You have already predicted the success of this book. I believe you are my number one fan.

Special thanks to Antoinette Coleman for her unconditional labor of love. If it were not for you, this book would not be in print. I love you, Toni, for being a wonderful and devoted friend, especially in supporting my dreams.

A Special Acknowledgment

TO THE FOLLOWING:

Mr. & Mrs. Bonner
Dr. Tusan Fregene, MD, and staff
Diana Gardner
Lisa Gardner
Ceilie Hall
Richard Jackson
Mr. & Mrs. Karam
Sheryl Newberry
Barbara Phillips
Beatrice Phillips
Druesillar "Dee" Rankins
Apostle Estes Ross
Anne Steele
Bob and Margie Taurianen
Fannetta Watson
The staff of Harris Adult School
The Harper Hospital oncology nursing staff
Karmanos Cancer Center
The staff of St. John Riverside Rehabilitation

I would like to thank these people for their support and special acts of kindness on my road to recovery. God bless you!

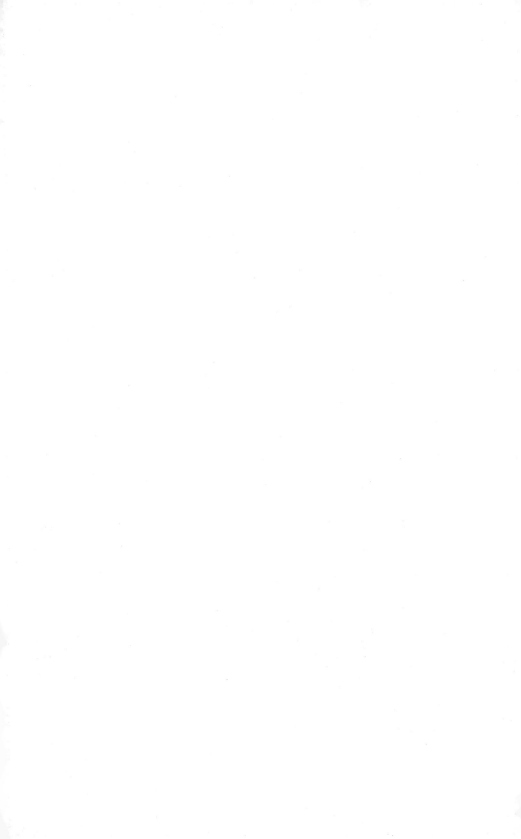

Introduction

We live in a time when life seemingly brings us challenges that we are so often not prepared for, and it invades our lives with a vengence. We cannot predict what the outcome will be, nor do we know how we will go through it. The only certainty we have is it will happen. It is called life!

At one of the happiest times in my life, I received a blow that changed it. There was no forewarning, and there was certainly not a team of solutions waiting to assist me with it. I basically had to go in fighting for my life against an enemy who had overtaken so many victims already. Who was I to think that I could battle against it and win? Who was I to think I had the courage to endure it? I was about to meet someone that I did not know existed. I had to come face-to-face with someone that was going to carry me through one of the most horrific challenges of my life. I had to come face-to-face with ME. I had to find out just what I was made of.

Unfortunately, we do not always get to choose our fate, especially those that so grossly affects our lives and our loved ones. If we could, I am sure that we would completely bypass them altogether. Therefore, I believe that God allows situations to bring to the surface our true character, which makes us better human beings.

When I was diagnosed with an insidious disease, I had no idea that it would provoke me to write this saga and the knowledge and life lessons I would learn from it. In fact, I did not even take before-and-after pictures because the last thing on my mind was to write a book. The only thing on my mind was to make it through each day and keep my household running, which was keeping the bills paid and food on the table.

During that time, I found out who my friends were and who was going to support me in my family. I did not care about a reading audience or if I could write a best seller. I was trying to do the hardest thing in my life at that time, and that was to LIVE! Therefore, who would have thought that I would even desire to write about my plight? For what reason? I am not famous. No one is knocking down my door, asking me to come and give my testimony. So, why am I telling you my story? Why did I feel compelled to write this book? So many other famous and well-known people in the world have experienced what I have gone through. They have also received big endorsements to tell their stories. So, who am I? These are the questions I asked God when He told me to write it.

The ordeal occurred in January of 1998, and I am just now telling my story. Oh, I tried to write it sooner, and I thought my manuscript was complete a long time ago, but I found myself having to stop because I had to add more or delete more. I had to constantly examine my motives for mentioning certain things. I had to make sure that what I said was correct to the best of my knowledge and recollection because I did not keep a journal. Remember, I was not trying to get a book out of the ordeal. Several times, God told me to stop writing because He did not want the reader to sense my bitterness. Yes, I experienced bitterness, and all I wanted to write about was my pain, but God would not let me; I had to let it go. He constantly repeated to me His profound words, "This is a comma in your life, not a period." Although it felt like my life was over, it really was just beginning. My destiny's path took on a completely new direction, and my life purpose became pronounced and profound. I believe that a near-death experience will do that for you.

So, why am I telling this story? Why did I write the book? It is for the many individuals who will experience life-changing events and may feel helpless and alone. It's for those who have a purpose and have not quite discovered it yet, and it is for those whose lives have given them nothing but lemons; I want to teach you how to make a lemon meringue pie and give everyone around you a piece of your sweet success and your recipe for overcoming your life's greatest challenges. Yes, that is right. This book is for you!

My ordeal was dealing with a sick body, yours might be the loss of a child (God forbid), the breakdown of a marriage, financial ruin, or just living your life aimlessly, not knowing why you are here, and trust me, that can be the worst experience of them all. Whatever it is that you are presently facing or what fate may bring your way, you are an overcomer, and your world is constantly changing for the better just for you. No matter what you face, always remember one thing, "This is a comma in your life, not a period." It is just a moment in your life; it is not the end. Whatever your challenge, you can finish strong and pass the baton of hope to others along the way. God bless you!

The Moment Of Truth

When I first met Dr. Souffront in May of 1997, I was the picture of health. I weighed over two hundred pounds, but I was well proportioned and solid. Of course, my mom always complained about my weight because she was used to seeing me in a much smaller frame. For years, I wore a size 11/12, and then I was wearing a size 16/18. I still looked great because of my medium/large five-foot-seven-inch frame and was able to carry the weight very well.

It was a routine physical and my first time seeing a doctor in ten years, so I was quite anxious to get a checkup. That was because visiting doctors was not my favorite pastime. However, at this time in my life, I was becoming more health conscious. I was very serious about being a motivational speaker and an empowerment trainer. Therefore, I thought it would be important that I set an example for other women.

As I began to fill out the forms the nurse had given me, my mind was thinking back on the last time I had seen a doctor, which was not a very pleasant experience. It was my six-month Pap smear, and the doctor was very insensitive and very rough. The mere fact I decided to see a doctor again made me feel very proud of myself. My level of consciousness was making me more concerned about my health and overall well-being. I went down the list, checking "no" to the different items concerning my health. When I was finished, I returned the forms to the nurse and waited anxiously for her to call me.

While I was waiting, I began thinking about how well things were going in my life and how good I felt. I had just bought a brand new SUV, a '97 Jimmy. It was white, trimmed in gold; it was beautiful. I also had a new male friend. He was handsome, educated, and he had his own house and vehicle. That was certainly a plus for me, considering what I had been attracting in the past.

He and I started seeing each other on a regular basis, and I was very elated. Everything was grand! My life was full of joy and splendor. I was looking forward to enjoying the summer in my new vehicle and with my new friend. So, what could go wrong, right? I stayed preoccupied that day, dreaming about all the fun I hoped to have.

It appeared to take forever for the nurse to call my name. All I could think about was who the doctor was that would have the privilege of examining me and giving me a clean bill of health. Soon, I heard my name called.

"Ms. Ford," the nurse said.

I got up and followed her to the back. She weighed me, measured my height, and took my blood pressure and temperature. Afterward, I was taken to an examining room and instructed to remove my clothes from the waist up. I waited for the doctor to come in, anticipating what he would look like because this would be my first time seeing him. I wondered if he would be someone with whom I could talk to freely and develop a rapport. At that time in my life, having a relationship with my doctor was very important to me. I was tired of changing doctors and having to start over again. As my mind was wondering, I heard a knock at the door, and in walked a brown-skinned, brawny man with beautiful white hair. He spoke with an accent and greeted me very pleasantly.

"I am Dr. Souffront," he told me. "So, what are you here to see me about?" This was the first question he asked me.

I explained to him how I had not had a physical in years, and it was time to do something about that. I was feeling good, and I desired to keep it that way.

Dr. Souffront began to ask me a series of routine questions about my family medical history. I recall telling him that my mother was a diabetic and my father had died of cancer (Hodgkin's) twenty years ago. After I answered his questions, he then began the examination, which only took place from the waist up. I remember how impressed he was with me. He kept saying, I looked like the picture of health and everything looked great at that point. After the examination, he instructed me to go to the nurse's station for my blood work and that would have concluded my complete physical. I told the doctor good-bye, and I truly thought that would be the last time I would see him until next year.

My life was normal for the next few weeks; nothing out of the ordinary was going on. There were no aches or pains at that time, but I did find out that my hemoglobin count was exceptionally low for my weight and size. Dr. Souffront was very concerned about the low count. So, he prescribed iron tablets and a B12 shot to help increase my blood count. He scheduled me to come back in a couple of weeks to discuss the results of my blood test and to see if my blood count had increased.

Between the time of our first meeting and the third visit, I started experiencing severe pains in my chest between my upper back and my rib cage. Isn't it amazing how all of a sudden your body starts falling apart after you see the doctor? It never fails. Before meeting the doctor, I was in no discomfort. When I saw the doctor again, I told him about the pains I was experiencing. He was sure that the pain was because of my anemia and did not appear to be alarmed about it. At first, I was not either because the pain came around and during my menstrual cycle, and it stopped after my cycle was over. Therefore, the pain would come and go. I thought because of the anemia, my body was lacking the proper amount of oxygen my muscles needed. This was very common among the women in my family.

A month went by, and the pains became more and more unbearable. In fact, the pain was excruciating and persistent. It felt like someone was standing on my chest. It was the month of June, and the pains were coming on a regular basis. I went back to see Dr. Souffront, and he scheduled more blood tests along with a chest x-ray and a stress test. This is where this story takes its turn.

My son had just graduated from high school, and he was getting ready to go to college that fall. Anyone who has ever sent a child to college knows how hectic preparation can be. It can be extremely stressful.

I wanted to give my son, Bayo, a graduation party, and because this was all new to me, I asked a few friends to help me plan the event. In the process of planning the party, I lost track of time. The stress test was given an appointed date, but the x-ray was to be a walk-in. The stress test was scheduled for the first week in July; around the time, we had that terrible tornado. I remember that day so well because the power went out in the hospital, and I was unable to complete my test. It was the day after the tornado that I had to go back to complete the testing. It was the Fourth of July, and I spent the early part of that day taking a test that ruled out any type of heart problem.

That day was over, and I anxiously waited for my son's graduation party to come and go. I was also busy teaching summer school that year and did not have a lot of time to rest.

The test results were in, and as I suspected, everything was normal. I knew there was nothing wrong with my heart. However, the pains continued to get worse. I knew there was something seriously wrong with me. The doctor got to the point of prescribing pain medication that did not help me. Now, remember, there was supposed to be an x-ray taken. It never happened because I was too busy. I became so busy that I just could not find a way to fit it into my schedule. So, eventually, I just forgot about it. The pain got worse, and I learned to live with it.

I began to tell everyone I encountered about the pains, especially my coworkers, because I spent most of my time around them. I was the youngest one at my work site. The other teachers were always teasing me about getting old. I was to turn thirty-nine that year on July 7, which was just a couple days away. They were always telling me about all the aches and pains that came with entering the forties. I would just laugh along with them as they continued to justify all the pain I was having. They did not always let on, but I suspected they were truly concerned about me. They were trying to spare me from any more anxiety than what I was already experiencing. No one wanted to believe I was seriously ill.

Continuous pain! Continuous pain! That was all I remembered going through for those next six months. It was driving me crazy, and it made me a regular visitor to the clinic and the emergency room. I recall leaving my job, twice, to go to emergency at Detroit Riverview Hospital. Going to hospitals was not one of my favorite pastimes, and that experience just confirmed all of my reservations.

During my first visit to the hospital, all they did was hook me up to an EKG machine to rule out anything being wrong with my heart. When the test confirmed that my heart was okay, they gave me a shot and something for heartburn. Then, they sent me home. The next visit to emergency was not any more productive. I could not understand why no one thought about taking an x-ray. As mentioned earlier, an x-ray referral was given to me in June. I failed to keep it because of my hectic schedule. I forgot about it; I really did! However, what was their excuse for not giving me one? I could not understand why I went to the hospital in pain, and I left in pain. It appeared to me as though no one was trying to find out what was wrong with me. Therefore, they ruled out my heart, but there was still pain in my chest and back. What was causing the pain? Why didn't anyone think about taking an x-ray?

The pain in my chest and back became my constant companion; I could look forward to it every day. From June until December, the pain was consistent, and it did not just stay in my upper body. Around the month of October, the pain started in my lower extremities. The pain was in my pelvic area, my hips, and my thighs. However, what was so strange about my condition was that the pain was never in my upper and my lower body at the same time. It was almost as though my body was having mercy on me and knew I would not have been able to tolerate the pain in both areas. When the pain was in my lower body, it would go from the left side to the right side; never would both sides hurt at the same time.

I cannot tell you which pain was worse. All I knew was that I was really beginning to worry, and I knew it was not old age that made me feel like that. I started making frequent visits to Dr. Souffront's office, and I cannot tell you that he was happy to see me. I was beginning to feel like he was not taking my complaints seriously. All he would do was give me pain medication. He did this twice. The pain medication never worked. It got to the point that the only thing that worked for me was over-the-counter Aleve.

Eventually, my body became immune to the pills, and I ended up doubling the dosage just to get some type of relief. What normally took a half an hour to work now took two hours. The constant discomfort was affecting every area of my life, and more than anything, my professional life was probably the most affected.

My job performance was steadily going down, and my coworkers did all they could to help me maintain some type of competency. I could not stand up and teach anymore. As a result, most of my days were spent sitting behind my desk, trying to stay as comfortable as I possibly could; and believe me, that was an extremely difficult task. I was going through hell, and I did not know what was going to happen to me. I knew that something was wrong with me, but the seriousness of my illness eluded me.

After many months of going back and forth to the hospital, and visiting my primary doctor, I began to feel quite helpless, and so did Dr. Souffront. My hemoglobin count was still extremely low, and this was causing my doctor to have a bigger concern than the pain that I had been experiencing. December 28, I was scheduled to see a specialist, a hematologist/oncologist. I was unable to keep my first appointment because something unexpected came up.

When I was finally able to keep my appointment with the doctor, I felt like that meeting would be my salvation. I knew that all my questions were going to be answered, but little did I know that there would be changes, possibly, for the rest of my life.

I sat patiently in the waiting room, unaware of the sickness that was all around me. I truly did not know that most of the people in my presence were gravely ill, and that I was about to become part of the fiasco. I found myself looking around the room at the many faces that stared back at me as if they were wondering to themselves which demon attacked my body and how long would I have to battle with it. They looked at me as though they knew something I did not know, and they already pitied me for it.

As I sat waiting to see the doctor, I thought about how the most difficult part of my suffering was my son having to see me in that condition. (This was before I was diagnosed.) He was home for the Christmas break, and I recall being in my upstairs bedroom in agony. He heard me in distress. When he came upstairs, there I was rolling on the bed, trying to find a comfortable position; there was none. I was moaning, and he did not know what to do. My son always looked at me as being a superwoman. Whatever the problem was, I could fix it. Therefore, when he saw me like that, it bothered him. He realized that I was not going to be able to make this problem go away. So, immediately, he began to pray for me. My son had never displayed this spiritual side to me before, and I was so proud of him. He recognized that only God would be able to help me get through that. He lay his hand on my back and began to pray a prayer for healing. In his helplessness, he left me and allowed me to get some rest.

I waited about forty minutes before my name was called. Then, a nurse came to escort me to an examination room. She took my weight and vital signs, then she told me to do what I hated doing: undress from the waist up. Know that I was suspicious. I was only there for my blood count. So, why was I being physically examined?

Well, this was the moment I was waiting for. Who would walk through the door? What would he look like? What kind of personality would he have? More importantly, would I like him?

"Hello, Ms. Ford," a tall, dark, and very handsome man spoke to me with an accent.

Immediately, I knew that he was from Nigeria and I also felt we were going to bond.

"My name is Dr. Fregene," he said. "So, what seems to be the problem?" He looked at the information that was sent over from Dr. Souffront's office concerning my blood count. I was about to find out why I had to remove my clothes from the waist up. After he looked at my chart, he started examining me, probing around my neck, under my arms, and around my pelvic area. He was looking for enlarged lymph nodes, and he found one. I have always said that if you look hard enough for something, you will find it, but that was one time I wished this was not true.

He found an enlarged lymph node near my collarbone, and he took my index finger, placed it on the lump, and told me to roll it around. It was about the size of a dime in diameter with a hump.

"This lump shouldn't be there!" he explained. "I want to find out what's going on with your body. After you get dressed, come to my office for your consultation."

By this time, I did not know what to think or how to feel, but I knew it was definitely time to be alarmed!

When I got to his office, I began to admire the artwork on the wall and the beautiful desk he had. I could tell this man had the same exquisite taste I had. He reminded me of my ex-husband, only he was much taller and heavier. Dr. Fregene came in about five minutes later, but it seemed like an eternity to me. My mind was wandering. I did not know what to expect.

When he sat down, I began to tell him about the pain I was experiencing in my chest area. At that time, he showed a lot of compassion. He really appeared to be concerned about what I was telling him.

"I want to have a biopsy performed, and I am certain that it will tell us what is going on inside of your chest," he stated.

Shortly after, I was scheduled to meet the surgeon, Dr. Mayben, who would examine me and explain the procedure. When I arrived at his office, I was in pain, and it was unbearable. When the nurse took me to the examining room, I could not even sit up. I was in tears, and I rolled around on the examining table to get relief. When the doctor came into the room, he could not examine me. I was so embarrassed that he had to see me like that. He did his best to console me and tell me about the procedure.

I was so happy to get out of there. I wanted to go home to get some rest. Aleve, here I come!

The biopsy was scheduled for January 26, and I was more than anxious about it. One of my friends, Alice White, accompanied me to the hospital for the operation. As usual, she and I engaged in laughter, determined that we were going to make the best of the ordeal. She stayed with me up to the time they wheeled me into the operating room.

This was it! I thought to myself. I was finally going to find out what was wrong with me. Oh, the excitement I felt was unbelievable. I had never had an operation before and did not quite know what to expect. I was not afraid, probably more curious than anything.

As they were entering the operating room, there was a picture of my chest x-ray hanging directly in front of me. Yes, they finally took an x-ray, and what I saw next caused me to understand there was something seriously wrong with me, and I was not too sure that I would have been able to handle it.

I recall asking the nurse, "Is that an x-ray of my chest?"

She replied, "Yes."

Suddenly, the last thing on my mind was laughing. I was told later that the mass in my chest was about nine centimeters in length. That is about the size of a large lemon.

They put me in a twilight sleep, the best sleep in the world. I could not tell you when they started or finished, but I was well rested. They took me to the recovery room, and Alice came in immediately to greet me. She was right there for me, and I told her how refreshed I felt.

Alice and I had only known each other for a short time, but we bonded immediately after we met. We were coworkers at Harris School, and she was the secretary of the head administrator when I met her. We began to spend a lot of time together. She would often accompany me to my doctor's appointments. In fact, she was there when I met Dr. Fregene. I did not know why at the time she was so willing to hang around me as I was going through this ordeal, but I later found out she was always making me laugh and keeping me in great spirits. We made a joke of everything; that was our way of handling the unknown.

I had to wait for about an hour before they released me to go home. Before the surgery, Alice helped me get prepared and waited with me until the time they came and took me for the biopsy. When I got back to my recovery bed, Alice was waiting for me with all smiles. Afterward, I was given instructions to call the surgeon in a couple of days for the results of the biopsy.

I could not rest for thinking about it. I did not know what to expect. I began counting the hours until it was time to phone the surgeon, Dr. Mayben. When I called him the first time, he was not available to speak to me. So, I waited until about three o'clock before I phoned him again. We finally spoke, and truthfully, I wished I had not spoken to him. What he told me that day would change my life forever, and my life's journey became an adventure for the next ten months and, possibly, for the rest of my life.

I asked him, "What were the results of the biopsy?"

He told me very insensitively, "YOU HAVE CANCER. You have Hodgkin's disease."

He gave me this information over the phone. I could not believe it! I repeated the words he said to me back to him to confirm if I heard him correctly.

"I HAVE CANCER?"

He said, "Yes." He told me to call Dr. Fregene, and he would discuss the prognosis and treatment with me.

"Okay!" I said, and I hung up the phone. As I sat in my living room in silence, my first thought was to call someone for sympathy and comfort, but

I could not move from my space. I was completely numb. I sat for hours in the silence of my home, not knowing what to think. All I could say was, "I have cancer," repeatedly.

The room suddenly became dark, and then silence gained a companion. I do not know how many hours I sat in the darkness and in the silence before I decided to call someone. However, the silence and the darkness were very much welcomed at that time because I did not want to hear anyone's voice or see anyone's face.

My sadness began to turn to anger, and I found myself crying profusely. The tears just would not stop. It was unfair to have cancer. I was not ready to die yet. I was not ready for this death sentence. What had I done to deserve this plight? In the midst of the silence and the darkness, I heard God speak to me in a still quiet voice, but I did not want to respond to Him. He spoke to me again, and I just surrendered and said, "Yes, Lord."

He then spoke to me the most comforting and profound words, "THIS IS A COMMA IN YOUR LIFE, NOT A PERIOD."

When He told me this, I began to embrace a peace that surpassed all understanding. I knew that I was about to go through the most horrific experience of my life, but I knew God would be with me. What I did not know was the lessons I would learn, and I had a great commission to share these lessons with others.

Did You Know?

The type of cancer I had was very rare (Hodgkin's disease). It accounts for less than 1 percent of all cases of cancer in this country. It is most often seen in young people aged fifteen to thirty-four and in people over the age of fifty-five. I was thirty-nine years old when I was diagnosed with the illness. Hodgkin's disease is a type of lymphoma. Lymphomas are cancers that develop in the lymphatic system, part of the body's immune system. The job of the lymphatic system is to help fight diseases and infection. Like all types of cancer, Hodgkin's disease affects the body's cells. Healthy cells grow, divide, and replace themselves in an orderly manner, which keeps the body in good repair. In Hodgkin's disease, cells in the lymphatic system grow abnormally and can spread to other organs. When the disease progresses, the body is less able to fight infection.

The estimated new cancer cases and deaths in the United States in 1997 were 7,500 estimated new cases and 1,480 estimated deaths (American Cancer Society Inc., 1997).

The Prognosis And Treatment

After sitting and meditating on the words that were spoken to me, I calmed down a bit and decided to make some phone calls. The first person I called was my sister, Diana. I believe I called her first because she was kept apprised of all of my doctor's appointments and every ache and pain I encountered. I felt it was only fair to tell her what the doctor told me. I remember hearing her on the other end of the phone, sounding stunned. She was at a loss for words, but I think she made herself say something for my sake.

"You are going to get through this," she told me, "and you are going to be just fine."

Diana always had something positive to say even in the worst situations. At that moment, I certainly appreciated her practice of positive thinking. I knew she was trying to be strong for me, but she was worried. She had never heard of Hodgkin's disease and had no idea what I was about to face or what my chances were for surviving it.

One thing about my sister I truly commend, she was not about to panic until she had all the facts. So, the next day, she got on the phone and spoke to a nurse she knew and asked her about Hodgkin's. When she was assured that I had a fighting chance of beating this beast, she was ready for the challenge, and she prepared me for it too.

After I spoke with Diana, I called Alice. She was so shocked; she did not know what to say to me. Believe me, neither one of us was laughing then. I was about to find out why Alice was placed in my life and the role she was about to play in my recovery. She comforted me with kind words and showed a lot of support. Then she revealed to me that she was a cancer survivor, not once, but twice. This was the first time she revealed this to me. All the time we spent together, I never knew this about her. She later told me that she wanted so badly for this not to be my fate, and bringing it up was not something she wanted to disclose unless she had to. She knew that the time had come and began to share with me her cancer experience.

Alice shared her experiences with me to give me hope and to let me know she was going to be with me all the way. She understood the trial and knew that I could not go through it alone. She was my anchor at that moment; I thanked God for allowing her to come into my life to walk with me as I traveled on the road of recovery and restoration. It was comforting to know that she would be with me.

When I finished talking to Alice, I sat in the dark for a while, wondering how I was going to accomplish the very difficult task of telling my mother. My mother lived in West Palm Beach, Forida, with my oldest sister. She was seventy-eight years old at the time; in fact, she had just turned seventy-eight years old that December. She was not very happy at the time for a number of reasons. When she left Detroit in July of 1997, shortly after a tornado virtually destroyed her neighborhood, she never thought she would ever see Detroit again.

My mother was a very strong woman, but her heart was broken because she had to leave her son William, who was in prison at the time. She just could not take the pressure anymore. She was so distraught about everything that was going on with him that she knew the best thing to do was to leave; leaving me behind saddened her too. I was her baby girl, and we were very close. If you had met my mother, she would have proudly told you that I was her "baby girl." She missed me a lot. Although she was in a beautiful city, she was very unhappy. She was going through her own private hell, and she felt trapped, not knowing how to get out. Later, she told me she had prayed that God would take her, and she often had thoughts of suicide.

I recall one day I had a conversation with a minister friend of mine who gave me a prophetic word. He told me that he saw my mother coming back to Detroit by either bus or train, but he could not tell me why she was coming.

Ironically, at that very time he revealed this to me, I was sick. God did not reveal my sickness to him though. I brought this up because I wanted to make a point. I strongly believe God heard my mother's prayer of despair, and He was about to give her a new beginning, and little did anyone know that that beginning would begin with me.

When I called West Palm Beach, my oldest sister, Marlene, answered the phone. We spoke casually, but I did not tell her what was going on. I was anxious to talk to my mother and get it over with. I did not know how she would react. Just the thought of her being more discouraged and unhappy was already eating away at me. I did not want to add to her pain, but I had to do it. She had to know.

My mind told me that if my mother was informed, then I could go through it. When I heard my mother's voice, my heart started pounding fast, and the first words I remember saying to her were, "Hello, Mom, how are you?"

She said, "Oh, I am all right."

Then I asked her if she was sitting down.

She replied, "Yes."

"Mom," I said. "I have cancer!"

The silence was so loud! I could not take it anymore. I did not know what she was going to say, but all she said was, "My baby, I am so sorry."

I felt relieved that the task was over, and I could get off the phone and get on with my life. We just made small talk after that because neither one of us knew what to say to the other. Finally, I got off the phone and sat alone with my two new companions, silence and darkness. We just hung out for a while.

The next day proved to be very interesting because I was experiencing some new symptoms. I was having blackouts. That morning, when I went to let my dog out, I passed out right at the side landing. When I regained consciousness, she was running around my reclined body. I cannot begin to tell you how long I was unconscious. As soon as I was able to get myself together, I prepared for work. It was very difficult to walk because it felt like the room was spinning around and around. I was not even sure how I was able to drive to work.

I slowly but carefully walked into the building and into the teachers' lounge. As the different instructors came into the room, I began to tell them the diagnosis. I was all right with telling everyone, but when my supervisor walked in, that's when the tears flowed.

Mrs. Vasteree Carter was the best supervisor I had ever had, and I enjoyed working with her and for her. I believe everyone did. I recall being able to go to her and just share with her what was on my heart. I even shared my dreams and aspirations. She would always encourage me and was supportive of whatever I wanted to do. So, it was extremely difficult telling her without crying. When I told her I had cancer, she began to cry, and that's when I started crying too. She hugged me and told me that I was going to get through it because I had too much to do and that ordeal was not about to take me out.

Telling my coworkers was very difficult for me to do because they all felt that it was something trivial. When they found out that it was cancer, they were shocked. I could tell they were trying to be strong for me, but it really took them for a loop. I was literally the youngest teacher in the building, and they all watched over me like mother hens. We worked so well together. We called ourselves the "Dream Team" because whenever we had a problem, we could always fix it. No matter how difficult the task appeared to be, we always rose to the occasion. Yes, working at Harris Adult School was very pleasant for me, and I thoroughly enjoyed it.

Finally, I was settled in my room for the morning and got my students situated with that day's lesson. I had a lot on my mind, as you could imagine. I tried hard to stay in good spirits for them. I did not want them feeling sorry for me because they would not have gotten any work done. Many of them were taking practice tests to prepare for their GED test.

I did tell them because they were very concerned about me. A few students were older than I was, and out of respect, I called them "Mom." We were a very close-knit class, and my relationship with my students was very special to me. There was nothing they would not have done for me. In fact, I recall over the summer, two of my students came to my house to help me plant flowers and elephant ears—I believe that was what they were called. We spent half the day together. It was so enjoyable. I had never planted anything before. Of course, I allowed them to do all the work.

I left my room to go to the restroom, and as I was walking down the hall, I felt very dizzy. My legs felt like they would give out at any moment. I found myself holding on to the walls for support. One of my coworkers noticed me and inquired to see if I was all right. I tried to play it off by telling her I was just a little tired and that I would be all right. Truly, I was scared; I did not know what was going on with my body. This was something new. I began to think about what happened to me earlier that morning when I blacked out.

When I got back to my classroom, I sat down at my desk with a sigh of relief. I made it! Trust me when I tell you that was a chore. I decided to phone Dr. Fregene to find out what would be the next plan of action. I wanted to know exactly what to expect, and I did not want it sugarcoated either.

He was very kind and appeared to be genuinely concerned about me. I felt comfortable with him, and I believed he felt comfortable with me. After all, he was going to play a very pertinent role in my life. I was glad that he was someone that I entrusted with my life.

"What's the prognosis, and what will the treatment consist of?" I asked him.

He told me, "You need to come to my office to discuss everything in detail." And then, he said, "I will do everything humanly possible to help you."

Those words were very comforting and reassuring to me, and I knew I was going to get through it. I began to hear the words that God spoke to me again, "THIS IS A COMMA IN YOUR LIFE, NOT A PERIOD."

I was about to begin my journey to Gethsemane, and I knew my cross was going to be heavy, but little did I know God was going to send some Simons.

Before I hung up the phone, a still, quiet voice spoke to me and told me to tell Dr. Fregene about the dizziness and numbness in my legs. So, casually, I mentioned it to him not knowing what to expect, but I certainly did not expect to hear what I heard.

He said to me in a firm voice, "Mrs. Ford, get off of the phone and get to emergency immediately!"

Now, I was getting nervous. I did not know

what to do. My mind was racing, and my heart was pounding fast. I could not think. Finally, I collected my nerves and called Ms. Freeman, one of my coworkers, and told her what the doctor said. She immediately came down to my room to help me get myself together. She notified Mrs. Carter to let her know she was taking me to the hospital and asked her to send a teacher to take over my room as I collected my belongings. Ms. Freeman was going to drive me to the hospital using my car. We asked one of my students to come along so Ms. Freeman would have a ride back to the school. We did not know what was going to happen.

When we got to Riverview Hospital, Ms. Freeman got me a wheelchair, and one of the guards wheeled me in while she parked my car. She and my student came in to find out what was going to happen with me. Would I be able to go home, or were they going to keep me? When I saw the nurse, I told her that I was diagnosed with Hodgkin's disease. I also told her my legs were feeling numb and that my doctor told me to come to emergency. They informed Ms. Freeman that they were going to notify my doctor, and they did not know how long the wait would be. So, I told her to leave me because there was nothing she could do for me and I would be all right.

She and my student left me there, and the wait seemed to be an eternity. Wouldn't you know it, of all the days to be at the hospital, I had to be there on what seemed to be the most crowded and busiest day of the year. They did not have any rooms available for me. So, they placed me in the hallway, and the wait was like being in the twilight zone. I felt like I was waiting forever.

FINALLY, a doctor came to see me. I must have been there for at least five to six hours. The school had already called the hospital to check up on me. Somehow, Alice found out, and she called the hospital too. I was bored and hungry. I could have lived with the boredom, but the hunger, NO WAY. Feed ME! I was becoming quite irritable and cold in that hallway.

They eventually put me in a room, and the doctor examined me. They also contacted Dr. Fregene, and he instructed them to give me an MRI. Now, Detroit Riverview did not have an MRI machine. For that reason, they transported me to Macomb MRI facility by ambulance. That was an experience because I had never ridden in an ambulance before. The attendants were very nice, and they were very empathetic. One of the attendants made me laugh to keep my spirits lifted.

When we arrived at the Macomb MRI facility, the attendant who made me laugh wheeled me in. I did not know what to expect. It was my first time having an MRI, and I have to admit, I had reservations about it. When I saw the machine, my reservations were confirmed. They were about to place me in a tube; at least, that is what it looked like to me. It reminded me of an old *Star Trek* episode I saw years ago when Spock died, and they launched his coffin into space. The MRI machine looked like a capsule to me.

I was placed on the MRI slab, and as my body began to enter the machine, I could feel my heart racing. As my head entered, literally, I lost my breath. I found myself gasping for air. I thought I was going to pass out. I hollered for the technicians to come and get me out of that machine. I could not believe it! I was claustrophobic. What a time to find out. There I was with a tumor in my chest, and only God knew what was going on with my legs. I discovered that I could not handle being inside of a machine that could possibly help save my life. They slid me out. One of the technicians told me that the test was necessary in order to find out what was causing the numbness in my legs.

Well, I was not hearing that at all. I let him know that this test was not about to happen unless they knocked me out! Unfortunately, they were not equipped for that procedure. So, they suggested to me that my face be covered with a towel.

"All right," I agreed, but I was still not a happy camper. I stayed in that capsule for about forty-five minutes, and that was forty-five minutes too long.

The test was finally over. The ambulance attendant came, placed me back on the stretcher, and prepared me for the ride back to Riverview. On the way back, I was not joking around and laughing because I was still trying to recover from the ordeal I had encountered. I knew the experience was going to leave an impression on me for a long time. I was right. I hate MRIs to this day.

When we got back to the hospital, shortly afterward, Dr. Fregene arrived. By that time, my sister and my niece arrived at the hospital. I called them earlier and left a message on the answering machine. They came and were very concerned about what was going on with me and even more concerned that I had to have a MRI.

They waited to see the doctor who was attending to me, but he had not gotten the results of the test back yet. So, he was unable to tell them what was wrong with me outside of what they already knew. I encouraged them to go to my house and see about my little girl, Daphne, who was my beautiful golden retriever mixed with white shepherd. She was my concern at the time.

I left her early that morning, and she had been in the house all that time. So, they left and went to attend to Daphne and my house. I was very relieved.

By that time, I had received several phone calls from coworkers and friends. A very close friend, at the time, also came to the hospital to see me. Lynn Ann, which was what I called her, but her name was Lynette. She popped up to make sure I was all right. I felt so special that so many people were concerned about me. She stayed with me until the doctor arrived, and, of course, we did what we always did: we laughed and told jokes. I believe she was afraid, but she did not want to disclose her feelings. She was trying to be strong for me, and I greatly appreciated her for that display of courage.

Finally, the results of the test were back. It was around 10:00 p.m. when Dr. Fregene arrived, and my stomach was about to start a riot because it thought I had forgotten about it. I was in the hospital emergency room for over ten hours, and I had not had anything to eat. I was starving! I could not understand for the life of me why no one was offering me any food, and God knows I was more than ready to eat. I may have been ill, but trust me, there was nothing wrong with my appetite and my taste buds.

The attending physician spoke with Dr. Fregene about the MRI results, and it was not a good report. This is where my story climaxes. Boy, when it rains, it pours. I was not expecting to hear the information that was about to be disclosed to me. I am glad I was already in the reclined position so I would not have too far to fall.

"Mrs. Ford, you have a tumor on your spine," Dr. Fregene said. "I am going to have you transported over to Harper Hospital where we can start treating you, immediately."

Was that a dream or what? A tumor was on my spine too. I could not believe it! What is going to happen to me now? I was dealing with many mixed emotions, and there was nothing I could do about them. I was frightened and confused because this was not supposed to be happening to me. I was supposed to be going forward in my life, not backward. All of a sudden, I was ill and did not have a clue as to how I was going to come out of this.

Oh yes! I believed in God, and I knew what he told me. I did not think for one minute about death. My only concern was time, how long was I going to have to go through that ordeal. My spirit man was at peace with all of that, but my mind was warring with it. I could not do that! I did not want to go through that. It was not fair! I did not deserve that. Just a few months before, I was happy with my life. I was working with a great team on my job, I had a new vehicle, I had a new friend, my son had left home to go to college, and I was getting ready to start living. Officially, I was going to start my nonprofit business and get my speaking engagements on the way. I was excited about life! Then, fate had to come and rain on my parade. What a bummer!

It took a lot of courage to accept the fact that I was going to battle with an insidious disease. Although God told me I was going to come through it, I still had to believe Him. I still had to apply my faith to what He said. Do not think because God gives you a word that faith does not have to be applied to it.

Trust me, if I had not stood in faith, I would have died. We can abort the Word with our actions and our words.

Consider it pure joy, my brothers, whenever you face trials of many kinds, because you know that the testing of your faith develops perseverance. But when he asks, he must believe and not doubt, because he who doubts is like a wave of the sea, blown and tossed by the wind. That man should not think he will receive anything from the Lord; he is a double-minded man, unstable in all he does (James 1:2-3, 6-8, NIV).

There were many times I turned my face to the wall and asked God to take me because it was getting unbearable, but the Holy Spirit reminded me of His intent and told me the choice was mine. I chose to stand because fulfilling the calling on my life greatly burned inside of me.

I was transported to Harper Hospital around midnight. I knew I had to begin preparing myself for the journey of a lifetime. Therefore, I asked God to lead the way. In spite of all I had to go through, I looked forward to one thing and one thing only, COMING OUT! As a good friend of mine would always say, "This too will pass."

After I was settled in my room, a team of doctors came in and surrounded my bed. Of course, Dr. Fregene was among them. I felt so special. There were about four doctors who came in to see me; they were all specialists.

There was a neurologist, neurosurgeon, radiologist, and oncologist. They began to talk among themselves. This conversation went on for about five minutes. Finally, Dr. Fregene spoke. He introduced the doctors and told me why they were all there. He explained that the tumor on my spine was causing them some concern, and they needed to decide whether an operation was required to prevent any further damage. The tumor was pressing against my spine on my lower back, and they were concerned about paralysis in my lower extremities. I was told I was in the fourth and last stage of the illness. If I was not treated immediately, I could lose control of my bowels, my bladder, and lower extremities, and possibly end up in a wheelchair for the rest of my life.

I began to pretend as if this was not happening to me. This was all a bad dream, and I was going to wake up any minute, but as they continued to talk, I realized I was not in the twilight zone. It was the real world, and it was my world. You have heard the expression that the whole world is a stage. Well, I was about to find out just how many actors were going to show up for the play.

The doctors decided to try chemotherapy and radiation therapy first to see how well the tumors would respond. If that did not do the trick, then they would have had to operate and remove the tumor surgically. That was, definitely, the last resort. They did not want to cut me because they felt it would cause a more serious condition.

All of the doctors left my room except Dr. Fregene. He hung around for another half an hour, and we sat around and made jokes. Oh, do not misunderstand me, Dr. Fregene took his work very seriously, but we had a special rapport. He knew I was very concerned, and that was his way of letting me know all was well. He even told me that the kind of cancer I had was curable, and he anticipated me being totally healed in about nine months. When he said that, I heard that still quiet voice say to me again, "THIS IS A COMMA IN YOUR LIFE, NOT A PERIOD!"

As I stated, Dr. Fregene took his work very seriously, especially when he had the pleasure of giving me a bone marrow biopsy. Dr. Fregene was not a surgeon, but you would have thought he believed he was when he took that long needle and placed it in both hip bones. I am not sure how long the needle was, but it appeared to be at least five inches long. The nurse cleaned the area with alcohol, and then he proceeded to do his thing. As he was pressing the needle into my hip bone, he had this mischievous look on his face. He was actually having fun doing this procedure. I knew that was the highlight of his day. Even now when I see him for my follow-up care, he teases me about it. The biopsy was performed to make sure cancer had not spread to my bone marrow. If it had, a bone marrow transplant would have had to be performed.

Praise God! There was no cancer in my bone marrow. So, he could go with the treatment as planned. Well, I was about to get ready to start on my journey. This was a journey that no one or nothing could have prepared me for, but as my father would always say, "I was going to come out, smelling like a rose."

A Rude Awakening

By the next day, most of my friends and family knew that I was in the hospital. My first week in the hospital, I received so many phone calls and visitors; I truly did not realize so many people cared about me. Sometimes, it was standing room only. I received many cards and flowers. I tell you the truth, a girl could have gotten used to that, I thought. I was also a model patient, and the nurses really enjoyed caring for me. I never complained or made a fuss about anything because my visitors kept me so preoccupied. When they left, I was exhausted and too tired. Many of the church members came to visit me too. So, my hospital stay was not a bad experience at all.

One of the most wonderful experiences

during my stay was when one of my coworkers, Ms. E. Singleton, came to visit me. This was a very significant event during my hospital stay because I never felt she cared for me. Our relationship was tolerable before I started having chest pains. I did not know why, but I just felt she did not care for me because of the different things she said about me. She never said anything to me face-to-face, but different people would tell me the things she would say about me. It was because of a man I was seeing, whom I later found out was not good for me at the time. She was quite opinionated about my relationship with him.

Ms. Singleton's visit was quite a surprise, but most welcomed. She did phone me to tell me that she was coming to visit me in the hospital, but I did not take it to heart.

When she entered my room, I was truly surprised but happy to see her. Trust me, when I tell you this, when you are confined to a hospital bed, you are happy to see even unexpected visitors. We started to laugh and talk about Harris School and what was going on in her personal life. The visit was very pleasant, but what she did next touched my heart. My legs and feet were ashy from a lack of attention. She proceeded to take some lotion out of her purse, and she began to massage it onto my feet and legs. It was the most humbling experience. In all the years that I have been in the world, no one had ever even offered to massage any part of my body.

At that moment, there was a spiritual bonding. This was the beginning of a healing between the two of us. I knew at that moment, she began to see a different person, and I saw a side of her that was warm and kind. Such a serene feeling came over me, and I knew that God was pleased with this union. Because of that spiritual bonding, when we see each other now, she treats me with admiration, affection, and respect.

I had so many unexpected visitors, two of which were my godparents, Bill and Minnie Tate. They arrived, demanding that I do something other than lay in that hospital bed. So, we went for a walk down the hall; Mom was on one side and Dad on the other. I knew that they were shocked to see me like that, but they did not talk about my illness. We just discussed what we were going to do when I got better. I had always shared my dreams and aspirations with them. Mom was the one who was instrumental in me getting a job with the Detroit Public Schools, and I knew she was not about to stop helping me now. They prayed for me and continued to do so even when I went home.

My treatment started immediately. The doctors decided that my radiation treatments be administered first. I was to have fifteen sessions, and I thought it was going to be a breeze for me. How bad could it be? It was like having an x-ray. They radiated my chest and abdominal area, which lasted for about twenty minutes. The procedure was not painful at all, but the treatments would continue even after I got out of the hospital.

Well, as I was getting used to all of this fine treatment, there was still something missing. There was still one person that I wanted to see but knew she would not be coming because I did not tell her I was ill. This was my friend, Dee (Druesillar). I did not call her because our relationship was always a roller-coaster ride even though we loved each other. We had known each other since we were eight years old. It was a very special bond between us, but many factors got in the way of our friendship. It was not fair to place blame on either one of us because that was just the way it was.

I had a conversation with my sister Diana. She asked me if I had called Dee.

I told her, "No! I am not going to call her." Dee and I had not seen or spoken to each other in about six to seven months. So, I was not about to call her to bother her with this. Yes, I missed her, but I was being stubborn, and I refused to call her.

Well, Diana had no problem calling her. Evidently, the news placed a flame in her heart. It was my fourth day there, and all my guests for that day had gone home. I was very tired, so I decided not to watch television, but just to get some rest. I was very restless that night and was beginning to feel some discomfort from the radiation. I was lying on my back when suddenly I saw a woman's form walk in my room. The form was silent, and as it stood at the foot of my bed, I watched it, and it did not move. Finally, I turned on the light, and I saw the most wonderful sight—my friend, DEE! There were tears running down her face, and when I saw them, I began to cry too. I do not know if she was angry with me or just elated to see me. She drove all the way from Wayne, Michigan, which would have been about forty-five minutes to an hour's drive to the hospital. It was past visiting hours, but no one stopped her from coming in to see me. That was truly a blessing. I knew then that everything was going to be all right. She visited with me for about an hour, and, of course, she scolded me for not calling her. Although she was happy that Diana called her, Dee felt the news should have come from me. She was right, and she got no argument from me.

Of course, she asked me about the prognosis, and she showed an interest for everything I was about to endure. After we talked about me, we began to catch up on her life. Somehow, the differences we had in the past seemed unimportant. I always said this about Dee, no matter what I was going through, she was always there. She was going to get there one way or another. She might have been angry as she was coming, but she was on her way. I could not ask for a better friend. No matter how bad the situation was, she always had a way of making me see that it was going to be all right. I did not know it at the time, but Dee was going to be one of my greatest comforts through the ordeal. As usual, she would just step right into her place. It seemed as though the people I least expected to be there came through for me, and those who I felt should have been there were not.

As I continue to express to you my saga, you will understand why in some instances this book was difficult for me to write. What I am about to disclose made me reluctant to write this chapter, but I knew I could not leave this chapter out. I was not ready to talk about this any sooner because it almost killed me, spiritually. The spiritual trial that I faced was more horrific than the cancer I had to battle. I tell people, this book should have been written first, but the spiritual and emotional pain that I faced was so grave that what you would have read would have been bitterness and resentment. I struggled for months about this book, waiting for the right time to write it, waiting for my emotional healing to take place, desperately hoping that I would still remember my experiences with the same fervency.

It is my sincere desire that this book be a blessing to everyone who reads it. I could not leave this part of the story out. People need to be aware of the struggles and responsibilities an ill person faces, and the role others should play in helping them get through it. Remember, every incident I experienced will convey to you instruction, inspiration, and a sense of hope in your life. I am sure you know that some life-changing experiences are not always comfortable to talk about, even after you have gone through them.

A major illness is something that I hope you will never have to face because like me, you will find out who is for you and who is not. Whom you can depend on, and whom you cannot. Who is genuinely willing to go all the way with you, and not just stop midstream. When a major crisis arises, it will tell you exactly what a person is made of. Remember, love and sacrifice may not always afford us the opportunity to have it take place at an ideal time when we want to help or spend our money. When we truly walk in love, convenience will not be an issue in our work of faith.

What good is it, my brothers; if a man claims to have faith but has no deeds? Can such faith save him? Suppose a brother or sister is without clothes and daily food. If one of you says to him, "God, I wish you well; keep warm and well fed," but does nothing about his physical needs, what good is it? In the same way, faith by itself, if it is not accompanied by action, is dead (James 2:14-17, NIV).

Now, my affliction was cancer, but your affliction may be something else. It could be a financial drought in your life, a broken relationship, or even misery in a present job or career. It does not matter what it is. God did not make man to be a Lone Ranger. He did not place us each on a deserted island to be alone, but instead, He made us sociable beings to be concerned and caring toward one another.

I believe people will not realize what it is like to be deathly ill until they have faced it themselves. Although I believed that God was going to deliver me from that plight, I suffered much despair because I looked for kindness and empathy from certain people only to be greatly disappointed. This experience was definitely a rude awakening! I strongly believe that if the shoe was on the other foot, I would have been honored to do whatever I could to make things easier. Now, allow me to share with you the traumatic experience I had and the people who played a major role in it.

My hospital stay had ended, and it was time for me to go home. I almost hated to leave. The treatment was so great, but I was tired of lying around and was anxious to see my little four-legged girl, Daphne. I knew she missed her mother greatly, and my sister and my niece were worn out from letting Daphne out several times a day and feeding her. I was aware of the sacrifice they made and appreciated it, but I was saddened when my mother later told me they complained about their gasoline usage; she paid them for their gasoline.

My sister always says, "We are family, and we should do what we can to help one another." Don't you think this was the perfect time to exercise that belief? I did not want to be sick, and I certainly did not want to inconvenience anyone. I felt my illness was a hindrance to my family because after I came home, I received very little assistance from them. I do not think they realized just how seriously ill I was and what all I had to endure.

I recall an incident that I experienced with my family. It was Mother's Day, and we had brunch at the St. Regis Hotel. My son, Bayo, was not home for summer break yet. Now I was still very ill and not quite halfway through my chemo treatments. I really did not want to go to brunch because I was still feeling very weak and tired, but my mother wanted me to get out of the house. I allowed her to persuade me to go, but I knew that I was not really up to it, and my pocketbook was hurting too. After we ate, it was time to pay the bill. My mother's portion was paid for because she was the matriarch of the family, but I had to pay for my own meal.

Now, some of you may be saying to yourselves, "What was wrong with that?" Nothing was wrong with that, but it would have been nice if they had been thoughtful enough to make that kind and wonderful gesture for me because I was ill and my son was not there to honor me. It would have made me feel special. My family likes to socialize and no matter what the occasion, especially when it is something pleasant, like birthdays, graduations, holidays, and retirement parties; but when there is a crisis, there is very little cohesiveness. What I found to be sad was that I do not even think they had a clue. If we were to have a discussion about this, they probably would not understand why I felt the way I did. I would like them to understand that there is more to being a family than just celebrating good times and attending to someone once they are dead. Families were created by God to forgo and be there for every situation, good or bad. I will say it again, if God wanted us to be alone, He would have placed us on an island to "fin" for ourselves and solely commune with Him. During this ordeal, I felt many of them just did not care about me. Some of my family members never even called me or visited me. Some came once, and I never saw them again until there was a special occasion. Maybe some of you, readers, may think I was just overly sensitive, and maybe I was, but I hope you do not have to go through a similar ordeal to find out if you would react and feel the same way. I personally needed to know that they cared, and I did not feel that they did. Oh, it was said with their mouths, but their actions proved differently.

Yes, it was time to go home and get back into living my life as normally as possible. My mother was scheduled to arrive in Detroit, the day before my discharge. She was coming to set things up so that I would be as comfortable as possible.

When I got home, a few people called to see how I was doing, but overall, it was a very quiet and lonely day. My mother was there, but she was more concerned with getting settled in and making sure everything was comfortable for me.

We watched television and talked about my illness. All she could say to me was, "I am so sorry, baby."

I did not really want to burden her with the responsibility of caring for me, but there was literally no one else that would have taken on such a task. I was practically immobile; I had to use a walker to get around. My 200-pound frame went down to 160 pounds. This all happened suddenly. The weight just fell off. My legs and thighs shook like Jell-O, and I walked bent over like an eighty-year-old woman. I definitely was not about to win a beauty contest. I became tired just walking from the living room to the bathroom. I found myself constantly out of breath. Oh, and by the way, those ten-hour workdays were just a memory because I was not about to see my job again for the next nine months. Therefore, you see, I was truly in bad shape.

The radiation was taking affect, and I began to feel miserable. The only thing I could do for myself was go to the bathroom and take a shower, and believe me, that was a chore. My mother had to do everything else. Remember, at that time, she was seventy-eight years old.

My radiation treatments continued when I went home. I was really beginning to feel the effects of the treatments. Swallowing became very painful, and I could barely eat solid foods. I was profusely salivating, all the time. My mouth would just fill up with saliva, and I had no control of it. I was miserable! The only things that brought me comfort were cold Gatorade chips. These treatments were actually burning the tumors. It was as if the tumors were being exposed to a microwave oven.

There were fifteen treatments scheduled for me. While I was in the hospital, I completed four treatments. So I had to continue the treatments while I was home. My insurance company arranged for an ambulatory service to take me to and from my treatments.

Now I want to share a wonderful story with you before I get into the reason for writing this chapter. Years ago, I had the opportunity to reunite with my biological brother, Cleva Watson, whom I met when he was only four years old. We were separated by fate. I cannot go into details about this story, but I always wondered where he was. I desired for him to know that he had a big sister who wanted to get to know him and be a part of his life. I prayed and asked God to allow our paths to cross somehow. Well, God answered that prayer, and we met. It was a miracle! I also discovered that he was not alone, but he did have an older sister that loved and cherished him. Her name was Fannetta Watson. She was a wonderful young woman I met through him over ten years before. At that time, I did not know this young woman would play such an awesome role in my recovery. She came back into my life in February of 1998. She appeared at my door to pick me up for my radiation treatments. When she rang the side doorbell, my mother opened the door, and I made my way to it in my wheelchair. When she saw me, immediately, she recognized me and I her. Neither one of us said anything at first, but I could tell she was taking special care with me. You may say that this was her job. I believe it was because I was her brother's sister.

She placed me on the lift of the ambulance and, very carefully and meticulously, wheeled me to an area to strap me in. Then, she helped my mother onto the van. My mother sat up front with her. At that point, she reminded me that we had met years before, and that she was my brother's sister, Fannetta. I was elated that I had an opportunity to see her again. Isn't it amazing how

God orchestrates things? Who would have thought that I would see her again under those circumstances? You see, although I met her and my brother almost ten years before, something happened to cause me and my brother to separate again. He did not know I was ill. She informed me that when she was given the assignment, she knew who I was. When she saw my name on the schedule for pickup, she could not believe it was me. I knew it bothered her greatly to see me like that. So, when she arrived at my home, she wanted to make sure I was who she thought I was. Her curiosity was confirmed.

Fannetta became my permanent driver for the duration of my radiation treatments, and although she did not have to, she made sure that she picked me up from my treatments and took me home. It was such a blessing to know that the person who was transporting me cared. She was always on time to pick me up and always on time to take me home. We got to know each other, and through this reuniting, my brother came back into my life, and until she passed away, my mother was close to his mother. Although I had someone to take me to my treatments, so many other areas in my life were lacking.

There were so many things I needed, and all

of a sudden, those needs seemed to come all at once. The plumbing in the house was going bad. I needed my lawn mowed. I could not drive, so we needed someone to take us to the grocery store and drive my mother to take care of business for me. *All of those people that visited me at the hospital, where are they now when I need them?* I thought to myself. I was beginning to see the big picture. This is why I entitled this chapter "A Rude Awakening." I struggled with this part I am about to disclose to you. My family in Detroit did not offer me much assistance, nor did my church. My family members were waiting on the church to do what they could do, and the church was expecting my family to help me.

I was becoming quite needy, and I hated it. Several weeks had gone by, and my ill bank with my job was almost depleted. I had to apply for assistance from FIA (Family Independence Agency). This was the procedure you had to follow in order to receive Social Security disability. I did not know how I was going to meet all of my financial responsibilities when my ill bank ran out, and I had very little money in my savings and checking accounts because I had to pinch off of them too. It certainly was not enough to get me through the duration of my illness. The Family

Independence Agency gave me less than $300 a month to live on. I also received $124 in food stamps. Here I was, a woman used to grossing over $3,000 a month starting to depend on $300 to meet my needs. I cannot lie. I was scared, and I felt helpless and all alone. My faith was definitely about to be tested. Not only did I have to believe God for my healing, but I had to trust Him big time to meet my needs too. My mother had needs, and it was important to me that her stay with me be as pleasant as I could possible make it under the circumstances. I knew it hurt her that I was struggling to pay the bills and provide for her, but I was determined I was going to do it, and God was going to help me in this great time of need. Now I want to get into why this book was so difficult to write, especially this chapter.

I was a faithful church member. I was a minister, I sang with the praise and worship team, and I was a faithful tither. My former pastor came to my home and told me to let him know what I needed. He also said that I had a church family who would do whatever they could to help me. I called my pastor several times to get assistance from the church, and not one time could he accommodate me. Oh, he did take me to emergency one day, but he was unable to take me home.

I did get visits from time to time from the first lady, but when she let me know that she did not appreciate me calling the pastor for assistance, I realized that those visits were just a formality. I believe the straw that broke the camel's back was when I asked the church for financial assistance. I suggested to the pastor that he take up an offering for me. I guess he resented that because it was my idea and not his. I truly meant no harm in asking.

At that point, I became the topic of discussion at the church. In fact, when I was taken to the hospital because of a very high fever, one of the members of the church came to see me at the hospital just to tell me how she felt about that gesture. I was extremely sick. My white blood cell count was extremely low to the point where it was life threatening. I had to be isolated from the other patients. She was not concerned about that. She came to "get me told" as she stated. I had no business suggesting that the church take up an offering for me. Just who did I think I was? Well, I was entirely too ill to speak in my defense at that time. I just lay there in my bed and allowed her to chastise me as she called it and humbly asked God to forgive me for the misunderstanding.

The pastor held a ministers' meeting to decide how to handle my situation. I guess the meeting was not in my favor. The pastor told me later that one of the more prominent families in the church strongly suggested that he not help me. I had to learn to trust God for my needs, and it was not the church's place to help me.

Defend the poor and fatherless: do justice to the afflicted and needy. Deliver the poor and needy: rid them out of the hand of the wicked (Psalms 82:3-4, NIV).

It is important that you understand that I was not expecting the church to take care of me, but I was expecting them to do more than they were doing. I just needed their assistance. I had many needs, and being a single woman, certainly, made it more difficult. I do not care what anyone thinks, but it is very difficult in this world when you are alone. I had to manage my home alone, and it was very difficult for me while I was ill. I just asked for some assistance. Many people in my church just thought I was asking for too much.

My mother cleaned the house, cooked, and accompanied me to all of my doctor's appointments and treatments. No one from the church offered to prepare a meal for us, help with the cleaning, or asked if I needed a ride to the doctor's appointments or treatments. If I called and asked one of my friends to prepare me something I had a taste for, they would, but it was nothing ongoing. Once a month the church had a women's meeting, and the ladies prepared a potluck. I felt that the first lady of the church could have organized the women to prepare a meal once a month just to take some of the pressure off my mother. Not even that was done.

When I joined that church one year prior to my illness, I felt so confident that the pastor and I made a connection. I thought we had a very good friendship; I felt very comfortable with him as my spiritual leader, and I thought he cared for my son, Bayo. I got along beautifully with everyone. I thought they cared about me. Therefore, when I became ill, I just knew that my church family would be there for me. I thought that when you were faithful to a ministry, it was the ministry's responsibility to help you in your time of need. I was not a benchwarmer; I was extremely active in the ministry. It was a rude awakening when I found out differently.

The pastor and I had a long talk one day when I came to service one Sunday. Service was over, I was on my walker, and I was going to my vehicle to go home when the pastor stopped me to speak to me. We stood next to my vehicle when he apologized for not being there for me. It was at that time that he informed me that one of the families of the church strongly suggested to him that he not help me because I was too needy, and they felt I was looking for a handout. I was deeply hurt by this information, and I asked him this question, "What did God tell you to do?"

There will always be poor people in the Land. Therefore I command you to be openhanded toward your brothers and toward the poor and needy in your land (Deuteronomy 15:11, NIV).

The poor are despised even by their neighbors, while the rich have many friends. It is a sin to despise one's neighbor; blessed are those who help the poor (Proverbs 14:20-21, NLT).

He could not answer this question. He only disappointedly looked at me and said again, "I am sorry."

I told him that I forgave him, and I went home.

Now I pondered on what he said to me, and I was so hurt that that family thought this about me. I could not help but think that maybe they were right. My adult life had been nothing but a struggle for me after my divorce. I struggled when I was married because my husband and I were newlyweds with a baby on the way and very poor. We were both still in college when we got married and our son was conceived. When I became single again, I struggled trying to raise my son alone, and I received little to no assistance from his father. I wondered if other people saw me as being a needy woman. I did not want to come across like that. I certainly did not mean to convey that image. I felt that I was so misunderstood. It was as if rejection followed me everywhere. I thought to myself, *So why should this situation be any different?*

I understand that it is human nature to be repelled from someone you think is always in your pocket. Therefore, it truly takes a compassionate, good-hearted, and spiritual person to recognize when someone is truly in need. Regardless of what they thought of me, I was extremely ill, and I was unable to take care of myself and all the needs that developed during this illness, and I was still entitled to mercy and compassion. At that time, I did not find it in that ministry. There was a lot of confusion that developed afterward because of "he said, she said." So, throughout the last six months of my ordeal, no one from that ministry called me to see how I was getting along. By the way, that family who suggested that I not be helped, I have forgiven them, and they no longer attend that church. I have also reconciled with my former pastor and his wife. It was years before I saw them again, but we have spoken and said our apologies and have gotten an understanding about the past situation.

Regardless of how people viewed me, as I stated before, there were still bills to pay, treatments to go to, and a house to maintain. In spite of the lack of assistance from my church and family, God still moved strongly on my behalf. He spoke to my heart and assured me that He was going to get me through this horrendous journey.

God touched the hearts of many other people such as my coworkers. They took up a collection for me—not one time, but three times. The first collections totaled almost $800. There were people from a former church, Agape Christian Center, who helped me. I attended there when my son was in junior high school. The Karam family came by, prayed for me, and gave me money for food. The Bonner family came by and was a tremendous blessing to me spiritually and financially. However, the people who blessed me in the greatest way were my friends Bob and Margie Taurianen. They came over one day, gave me Holy Communion, and months later paid my house note for the month of August. Margie helped clean my house. She also had her brother come in and install a brand-new toilet at my mother's request. None of those things did I ask them to do, they just did it from the goodness of their hearts. In spite of what others said about me, they did not shut up their bowels of compassion.

Many others were a blessing to me. I want to tell you about this one person in particular. Many of my students continued to keep in touch with me throughout my illness. One of those students was Benson. Benson was a very special student because he had a learning disability, but he proved to be one of my brightest students. During his childhood, he encountered several head injuries, so consequently, life was somewhat difficult for him. I understood him and tried to give him the encouragement he needed to get by. He called me often to see how I was doing, and we would talk.

During our sharing, I disclosed some difficulties I was having in several areas. He took it upon himself to introduce me to a minister friend of his, Apostle Estes Ross. Initially, we met over the phone, and this man immediately took me under his wing. He started calling me his little sister. He would pray for me and encourage me through my ordeal, and he even had a mini fund-raiser on my behalf. He was very caring; my mother liked him immediately. To this day, I still call him my big brother. I will never forget his kindness.

God sent a miracle. In fact, he sent several. He moved so miraculously that it was like watching a big-screen TV. I was afraid to blink because I thought I might miss something. Many people outside of my church and family gave me assistance. Some brought money to buy food. Some gave me money to take care of bills and living expenses. I was given spiritual tapes and books on healing. One of the couples that I mentioned earlier, the Bonners, bought me herbs to help with my healing.

Yes, God moved and continued to move, but I still struggled with seeing so many people, whom I thought cared, do very little or nothing. I just could not get my mind off of it. As I mentioned previously, many of my family members did very little or nothing to assist me during this time. I believe that they just did not want to get involved. Maybe they were afraid they would have to do too much and that would interfere with their lifestyles.

Now, some of you may be thinking to yourselves maybe they did not know what I needed.

Well, let me tell you my response to that assumption, ASK! I could not believe that they could be so insensitive. Although many people helped me, I needed to see my family get more involved. I needed to feel like they cared. A phone conversation, a drive to let the breeze blow across my face, a visit with a lengthy conversation, these were the courtesies I was looking for.

At that time, my sister was getting ready to retire, and her daughter was planning her retirement party. Her mind was solely on her upcoming event. This did not surprise me because she had always been like that. She would come over to the house, kiss me on my forehead while I was lying on the couch, ask me how I was doing, and then go into the kitchen to talk to my mother about her retirement party. I believe she was also planning on buying a new car. I understood her excitement about her party. She worked hard for many years, and it was time for her to start enjoying life. Nevertheless, not once did she ever take the time to have a meaningful conversation with me during one of her visits. She would go into the kitchen and share all the wonderful things that were happening in her life with my mother. I cannot remember a time she asked if we needed anything or how we were getting along in terms of the needs in the house. In fact, none of my family members, who lived locally, showed any real concern. Please understand, again I did not expect them to take care of me or go into debt because of me, but I was looking for more empathy than I received, especially for my mother. I knew not to expect anything for myself. Later, I did learn that my sister gave our mother a few dollars from time to time, and I was grateful for that.

She always said that she did not have any money to help anyone. She worked hard for her money and did not feel she should have to share it with anyone. Therefore, I imagined this was why she seldom offered. If everyone felt like her, there would be no compassion in the world, and many people would be lost for the lack of help. I thank God that some people recognize the power of giving and meeting the needs of others. I struggled with this for many days and months afterward. I became very bitter, and I asked God to forgive me and allow me to get past this. I supposed my sister did not realize how much we needed her; therefore, I have forgiven her.

As I continue to walk back down memory lane, I think back on the conversation I had with my brother, Craig. This was at my brother William's funeral. I asked him why he did not come to visit me while I was ill. He told me that he knew how I was doing because Diana gave him progress reports. Now, for some reason, he thought that was cute or funny because he laughed about it. Well, let me tell you, I did not care for that explanation at all. He visited me one time in the hospital, and that was the last time I saw or heard from him until my brother's funeral a few years later. This bothered me because I grew up with him. We were a year apart, and I thought we were closer than the behavior he displayed. I expected him to call and come to see me, and there was no excuse acceptable to me from him. I learned that he did not come around because he was angry with my mother for accusing him of something he says he did not do.

Trust me, what she accused him of, he had often done in the past. So, he earned the blame. Regardless of that, he should have been there for his sister. I was gravely saddened by his decision not to come around, and my mother was hurt too. I could never understand why he would have allowed anything to stop him from being there for me.

When I reflect back on the whole ordeal, I believe that my family and church did not respond to me properly because they took for granted that my seventy-eight-year-old mother could and would handle everything. If you asked me, that was even more reason why they should have gotten more involved. She was old!

Again, this book should have been written first; but because of pain and disappointment, I was not psychologically, emotionally, and spiritually fit to do it. Also, there were lessons I had to learn from these experiences. So, I asked myself, "Tunishai, what did you learn from this experience?" I learned firsthand that God will move with or without man. I learned that it's human nature to be selfish and self-centered, especially, when we are expected to go into our pockets and use our own resources to help someone else. It is only by the Spirit of God that a person can be unselfish and giving during times of need. Therefore, I learned to place my trust in God and not look to man because as long as man is led by his flesh and not the Spirit of God, he cannot understand the significance of giving and caring fully. I also learned that everyone should have some type of disability insurance in place, especially, if you are employed and it is offered.

While you are in good health, you need to take responsibility for unexpected occurrences or you can end up as I did, at the mercy of other people. I was bitter for a long time and in need of inner healing for my emotions. I realized that people are not always going to respond to you the way they should, but this did not interfere with my caring for others. When I finally got that revelation, I was able to start on this book and write this chapter.

"Remember, love and sacrifice may not always afford us the opportunity to have it take place at an ideal time when we want to help or spend our money. When we truly walk in love, convenience will not be an issue in our work of faith."

It took me nine years to do it. My anniversary for being cancer free for nine years was August 2007. I want people to understand the plight of having an insidious disease and the importance of others becoming actively involved in the recovery from that illness. An ill person is dealing with far more than just the physical aspect of the illness.

They are affected spiritually, emotionally, psychologically, and financially. Unless you go through a major illness, you can never understand the reality of the plight. Through sharing with you my experience, I hope that a greater empathy will be instilled in your hearts for your loved ones, and that your love can be channeled for those who are suffering. Get involved! Do not assume that an ill person has certain things in place. Do not let the responsibility be solely placed on one person. Ask what is needed. It might just be a friendly conversation or a nice long drive just to feel the wind on his or her face. You do not know when you may need support from others. When you help, you are planting seeds for you and your loved ones. God, looking down, will reward you for your kindness.

No one could have told me that I was going to have cancer. It snuck up on me. I would not wish this on anyone, but statistically, around 33 percent of the American population has had cancer. That number is growing and will continue to grow. You have to ask yourself how far you want to go with your involvement with someone who is ill because you may never know when an illness will come upon you. You may need someone to "GO ALL THE WAY!" The principle is that if you sow good seed, it will surely come back to you. Likewise, the same is true if you do not sow seed at all, then you have nothing coming back. Remember, when you least expect tragedy or hardship to come, it will. Ask yourself if you were there for someone during his or her time of need. If you were, rest assure that someone will be there for you.

Do not be deceived: God cannot be mocked. A man reaps what he sows. The one who sows to please his sinful nature, from that nature will reap destruction; the one who sows to please the Spirit, from the Spirit will reap eternal life (Galatians 6:7-8, NIV).

God wants us to be concerned about our brothers and sisters. He wants us to have an active role in each other's lives, and not be so passive when we see them going through their trials or hardships. Prayer is not always enough. We should know that faith requires us doing, if we have the ability to do for our brothers and sisters. It is called hypocrisy if we do not act in faith (James 2:15-17).

God Hears A Mother's Prayer

During my illness, every day was a challenge for me. I never knew if I was going to be rushed to the hospital due to my white blood cell count being low or if I was going to have another day of depression. I had a rigid schedule. Every day, for fifteen days, I had radiation treatments to my chest and spine. A few weeks later, my chemotherapy started. Every other week, I was going to Dr. Fregene's office for my chemotherapy, and being extremely sick afterward was what I had to look forward to. I hated my life at that time. Many times, I asked God to take me because the ordeal was becoming unbearable. The treatment was worse than the disease. I did not know how much more I could take. It would take me days to start feeling better after the treatments and then it would begin again. I was certainly a basket case for the first few months.

My pillar of strength came from the most wonderful person I knew, my mother. She never gave up hope, and she was the perfect caregiver to me. I do not know what I would have done without her. She never complained, and no matter what the task, she was always up to it. Now, let me remind you again, she was seventy-eight years old. I believe God gave this little woman supernatural strength to do what she did. Moreover, it was during this time that I learned that my mother was truly a spiritual woman and had a direct pipeline with God.

Every morning, without fail, she would pray around five o'clock. She had certain scriptures she read, but what blessed me the most was when I would see her put her frail but very beautiful hands together and pray and ask God not to take her baby girl! She would tell Him that she was not ready to let me go, and she would remind Him of how she prayed five years for my birth, and that I had a great calling on my life that I had to fulfill. This faithfully took place every morning for the entire duration of my illness. She was a woman who could not tell you where a scripture was found, and probably if she could, she would misquote it, but she believed that God could do anything but fail. She prayed a fervent prayer from her heart and was consistent. I have never seen such diligence, have you?

Continue in prayer, and watch in the same with thanksgiving (Colossians 4:2, KJV).

My voice shalt thou hear in the morning, O lord; in the morning will I direct my prayer unto thee, and will look up (Psalms 4:3, KJV).

My mother would get up every morning, prepare breakfast, and make sure I had my meds. When it was time to pay the bills, she would handle that, and when people gave to me in any manner, she would write the most thoughtful words to them in the thank-you cards. I gave my mother and my niece power of attorney of me in case things took a turn for the worse. She took care of all of my business according to my instructions, of course, and everything began to fall in place.

My mother needed money for her personal needs. When she prayed and asked God for extra money to come into the house, God answered her prayer in a big way. A friend told me about applying for money for my mother because she was my caregiver. I called FIA, and they immediately took care of the paperwork. My mother started receiving money for taking care of me. When my ill bank ran out from my job, my mother petitioned God again. He touched the heart of a former coworker, Ceilie Hall, to go back to the elementary school I was assigned to years ago and take up a collection for me. A few days later, she brought me an envelope full of money. It was over two hundred dollars!

Now, I do not want you to get the impression that I did not pray. I did pray daily, but I believe that my mother's prayers touched and moved God. It was at that time in her life that God was working something out in her. He wanted her to know that He was with her too, even in that dark hour. You see, not only was God preparing me for a miracle, He had one for my mother also. My mother needed to be reassured at that time that God was with her because of all she went through. It was not my circumstance that brought my mother back to Detroit. God heard a previous prayer that compelled Him to move in her life.

In July of 1997, Detroit was hit by a terrible tornado. If you are a Detroiter, I know you remember the event all too well. My mother's house was not touched, but some of the surrounding homes in the neighborhood were destroyed or damaged very badly. My mother was facing legal matters that concerned my brother William, and the whole ordeal was draining her. She just wanted to escape from all of those legal matters. When the tornado happened, that helped her make up her mind. My oldest sister, Marlene, talked Mother into moving to West Palm Beach, Florida, to live with her and her dad, my mother's former husband. My mother accepted the offer and sold her home for little or nothing to get out of Detroit.

Although Mother was gone, and I was very lonely for her as she was for me, I did not want to do or say anything to persuade her to come back. At the time, I felt the move was good for her. My mother ended up being very miserable down in Florida. She did not have a life because my sister had too much control. Mother told me later that she asked God to take her, or she was going to commit suicide. She was so unhappy. She was not getting along with her former husband, and she did not like being bored. Mother was used to being active. She was very involved in social events when she lived in Detroit. My mother would cry out to God and ask for deliverance. Little did she know God was getting ready to answer her prayer.

I recall one day, I went to visit a minister

friend of mine who was greatly used in the prophetic gift. We were engaged in a conversation when suddenly he said to me, "I see your mother coming back to Detroit, either by train or bus."

I did not understand because I knew that my mother really had no reason to come back. I did not worry about it; I just placed it in the back of my mind. Now, the ironic thing about this event was that when he told me this, I had cancer. God never revealed that to him. He just showed him that my mother would be making a trip back to Detroit, but he did not know why. When I think back on this, I give God the glory because He was working out a bigger blessing. He was going to use my ordeal to bring my mother peace.

Although I was very ill, my mother was at peace. She and I beautifully got along. We enjoyed each other, and I believe that my mother found a new purpose for living. She felt useful, needed, and appreciated. My mother was happy. She did not want to see me sick, but she would not have thought about coming back to Detroit. She would have just stayed in Florida and remained unhappy, but God said, "Not so!"

She actually had what I call a rebirth. You have heard the old cliché, "God works in mysterious ways." He was about to kill two birds with one stone by performing a miracle for two people, who were so desperately in need of one another.

Each day that went by, I could actually see myself progressing, and Mother never doubted that I would. She just continued to pray for me and go about her daily routine of caring for me. I have to admit, I really enjoyed the pampering. It certainly bonded us closer together. We did everything together, and I looked forward to spending time with her. We had not always been able to share that kind of quality time together. Even when I was growing up, we were never that close. My mother was always preoccupied with the cares of the world and did not have the energy to give me the emotional stroking that I needed. I do not fault her for that because I understand now what she was going through. However, she was an excellent provider and teacher. She always found time to teach us about everything she learned from measurements to sex education. She even taught me about God.

As a small child, she literally taught me about God on her lap. She would tell me Bible stories and how to pray for God's blessings. I must say, at a very young age, I had a relationship with God. I attribute this to my mother's strong faith in God and her overall example of being a good person. I loved her with all my heart, but we never had the closeness I desired until that time in my life. Maybe, it was because she truly had nothing else to be concerned about. She was old and tired of the drama that came with life, and the only fight she had left in her was the fight to see me recover from that disease.

My mother was fighting for my life, and that was the greatest gift she could have given me besides making the ultimate sacrifice of giving birth to me. She was unselfish, and at this time in our lives, nothing else mattered.

My mother's attentiveness prevented me from almost dying because I came very close to it. One evening, I was resting after my chemo treatment, and Mother was taking my temperature
every hour on the hour. It was really getting on my nerves! She was a regular little nurse; she would follow the doctor's instructions to the letter. Well, this particular time when she was taking my temperature, it went up to 103, and my mother was frantic. I personally did not care and just wanted to be left alone. I was very stubborn about going to the hospital, but Mother was insistent. I was rushed to the hospital, and they immediately placed me in isolation. My white blood cell count was low, which meant my immune system was not going to fight off

germs very well. I had to have a blood transfusion that would take a few days because they could not find my blood type.

When people came into my room to visit me, they had to wear a mask and gloves in addition to washing their hands. I knew that it was very serious because in order to get to my bed, you had to walk down a corridor. The next morning, the attending doctor told my mother and niece that if they had not gotten me there when they did, I would have died within twenty-four hours. There were other episodes like that where I had to go to emergency, but somehow, I always got there in the nick of time.

I strongly believe, in fact, I know that it was all because of the prayers of my mother and others that caused intervention to take place. I know my mother had found favor with God. She was not perfect, but her heart was pure and her integrity impeccable. She would help anyone that needed assistance. I know that this was her special gift to the world, and she was a special gift to the world. I have found no other woman that could fill her shoes. There was no greater hero, and no one can take the place that she holds in my heart. I know that my mother was God's special one, and whatever her heart's desire, He granted it because her love was an unselfish love.

When a mother cried out to Him for her child, He heard it, and the blessings that availed were unlimited. I do not know if you can say the same about your mother, but if she's alive today, and you are reading these words and digesting them, I want you to tell her just how much she means to you, and then praise God for giving you a special gift in the form of your mother. My mother was my inspiration. If it were not for her, I do not know what I would have done. No one would have been willing to make the sacrifice that she made. If she had not come or if she was deceased at that time, I would have ended up in a nursing home because I do not believe anyone else would have been willing to step up to the plate to help in that capacity. My mother was my hero. She was, indeed, the WIND BENEATH MY WINGS!

That was almost fifteen years ago that my mother, literally, nursed me back to health, and I will be forever in her debt. I pray that my mother is smiling down on me, knowing that this book will be a blessing to many, many people. I pray she is pleased with what I have become and what I will yet become. I am a stronger and better person today because of having known her. When I look in the mirror, I see her dreams in my eyes, and my thoughts are forever striving to fulfill her vision for me.

My mother died on April 4, 2006. She was eighty-five years old. I prayed with her the night before, and she was dead early the next morning. I miss my mom, and it is hard to believe she is gone. I cannot imagine going through the rest of my life without her. My tribute to her will be this book and every other book I write and to live my life to the fullest and become the woman that she prayed God would allow me to become.

The eyes of the LORD are on the righteous and his ears are attentive to their cry (Psalms 34:15, NIV).

An Angel Named Tee

The chemo treatments were becoming unbearable; I hated going to get them. Just the thought of going to the clinic made me sick. I could actually taste the chemo in my mouth and smell it in my pores. I did not think I was going to make it. My body began to break down every time I had a treatment, and this caused Dr. Fregene great concern. Although I was halfway through the treatments, I did not want to see another needle, and I certainly was not looking forward to the nurse placing that hooked needle in my Mediport (a small medical port surgically inserted into the patient's body so medicines can be administered). I just wanted it to be finished.

I had to take a medication called Neopogen because my white blood cell count was always low after my treatments. My insurance did not want to pay for the real stuff. They wanted to give me the generic brand, but Dr. Fregene insisted that they pay for the good stuff, which was $1,500 per box. If I recall correctly, there were only ten vials in a box, or there may have been less. I know they were glad when I got better; they probably had a party to celebrate (smile).

To ensure that the medication was administered correctly, they assigned a nurse to come out to the house and administer a shot to keep my white blood cell count normal. I really appreciated that because that meant my mother would not have to do it. My mom would have tried to do it, and I am sure she would have done a fine job. But let's face it, my mother was not a nurse, and she had enough to do already.

I recall the first day that I met that special lady. It was a beautiful sunny day, and the temperature was perfect outside. I remember it was just before Easter, the birds were singing, and the tree branches were doing their usual dance to the cool breeze of the day. It was an early Monday morning when the doorbell rang. My mom went to the door to see who it was, and on the other side of the door stood a petite dark-skinned woman with a wonderful smile, and she carried a briefcase. My mother liked her immediately because she could see that she was going to be a tremendous blessing to us. Mom was right.

God sent someone who was kind and understanding to help me. You are probably wondering what made her so special. Well, she listened to me, and she was concerned about my pain. Not just the physical pain, but the emotional and psychological too. She often overstayed her time to give me extra encouragement. We would talk about how God was healing me and sustaining me during that very difficult time in my life. She even brought me small gifts just to cheer me up. To this day, I am sure she was unaware of how much she blessed my life and took so much pressure off my mother.

Nurse Tee, as I called her, wanted my mother to learn how to administer the shot just in case she could not come by to do it. Mother was a little nervous about that, but she paid attention as Nurse Tee demonstrated on an orange. Mom had to do it a couple of times, and I must tell you that she had a heavy hand, and it hurt. Well, after I complained so much, Nurse Tee decided that she would not leave this task to my mother. So, she made it her business to be available to give me the shot.

It was Easter morning when Nurse Tee was

on her way to church. She was running late, so I just knew she was not going to make it. I prepared myself for the worst. Yep, you guessed it, Mom would have to give me the shot. I was not looking forward to that. Just as my mother was about to stick me, the doorbell rang, and I went to the door to see who it was. It was the most wonderful event of the day. There was an angel at the door, an angel named Tee. She came to give me my shot, and I had tears in my eyes, not because she was going to give me the shot, but because she thought enough of me to come. She was running late for church, but I was important to her. She showed me there was still empathy in the world, and I was worthy of a little of it. She was off on Easter Sunday. She did not have to come to my house; she was not being paid for that day, nor did her job know about it. That event impressed me so much.

When she left, I just sat on my couch and thanked God for the blessing that He gave me through this wonderful and magnificent person. I knew that He was sending me many special people, and she was one of them. It is not every day that you meet someone who is willing to show kindness without getting something in return or allowing himself or herself to get so involved with someone, even when it is not a close friend or relative. She only had a few more times to come to my home to administer the shot. When she finished her assignment, I never saw her again, but she left me with the memory of being a very special person. Because we live in a very apathetic world, it matters when someone goes out of his or her way to care.

You may be wondering why we did not stay in touch. Well, she was my angel only for that time in my life. She finished her course with me, and that was it. I realized that she was not going to be a long-term friend, and I was fine with that. Do not force what is not meant to be. People are sent into our lives for different reasons. Some will pass through it, and others will stay longer. Be grateful that essence was given to you. Truly, I was blessed to have an angel named Tee. I will imagine she is out there, somewhere, brightening the life of someone else, just simply doing what she does best. Nurse Tee, wherever you are, God bless you!

Be devoted to one another in brotherly love. Honor one another above yourselves (Romans 12:10, NIV).

Vernetta's Song

During the spring of 1997, I was riding high on life. Everything was perfect for me. I loved my job because I worked with a wonderful team of people, and every area of my life was fulfilling. I had just gotten a brand-new gold-and-white 1997 Jimmy SUV. It was wonderful! I had a new man in my life, my son was graduating from high school and getting ready for college, and I had a wonderful prayer partner and friend named Vernetta who always helped me keep things in perspective. Vernetta played a very pivotal role, but little did I know the impact she would have on my life.

Vernetta was like a beautiful flower in the midst of cactus plants because she was so radiant and nothing ever seemed to disturb her peace. She was good for me, although I often wondered if I was good for her. I was the one always seeing the negative in a situation, but Vernetta was the one who was always able to point out the good. Even when I was not very desirable in my actions, she never rejected me. Oh, she was truly a gem.

When I decided to go on this health kick, I shared it with her, and we decided we would go on a diet together. You will recall I had not had a physical in over ten years. She encouraged me to go and have one. We spent a lot of time together over the phone because as I stated earlier she was my prayer partner. We prayed every Tuesday evening around eight. She was very gifted, and God would show her things. Some would call her a seer. Oh, she loved the Lord and always acknowledged the Holy Spirit as the one working through her. I trusted her, and whatever she told me usually happened.

I recall when there was a major layoff about to happen within Adult Education. I was on the list. I saw my name on the list at a union meeting. I went to Vernetta very upset, and we prayed about it. I did not know what was going to happen to me. Vernetta prayed for me and got quiet so that the Holy Spirit could speak to her. She confidently told me that she did not see me losing my job. I had to challenge her, of course, because again as I stated earlier, I saw the layoff list. She was insistent that I was not going to be laid off.

A few days later, while I was sitting at my desk, I received a phone call from a woman I did not know. She told me that a very important meeting was going to be held concerning the layoff. She insisted that I come to support the meeting. I was hesitant, but I heard that still quiet voice as clear as my own thoughts saying to me, "GO!"

I went to the meeting after work. For some reason, I had a hard time finding the church where the meeting was to be held. When I finally arrived there, I was about fifteen minutes late. I recall walking into the room, and every chair was filled with disgruntled people. Quietly, I sat down in the first empty seat I could find, and someone handed me a list of names. I examined it very closely. It was the final layoff list. It was in alphabetical order. I allowed my eyes to closely scrutinize the list. When I got to the *F*s, I did not see my name. I could not believe it! I looked again to make sure my eyes were not playing tricks on me. My name was not on the list. I sat there in silence. All I could do was silently praise God. I could not wait to get to Vernetta's house. When I left the meeting, immediately, I went to her house. I was so happy!

"Vernetta, you were right!" I shouted. "I didn't get laid off."

All she said with a grin on her face was, "I told you that you would not get laid off." Vernetta was right about many other events in my life too. Unfortunately, though, she did not see what was going to change both of our lives forever.

After I went for my physical, a few weeks later, I started have excruciating pains in my chest. I often shared this with Vernetta. These pains went on for months. At the same time I was going through a physical challenge, Vernetta was also experiencing pain in her lower back. Now, because she was overweight, she felt it was due to the weight. She started seeing a chiropractor for treatments. It did not offer her any relief. Often, I found myself having to go over to her house just to talk to her because she did not feel up to talking on the phone. I would go and have to bang on the door several times before anyone would come to the door. She lived with her son and daughter-in-law.

Finally, when I did see her, she was in a lot of discomfort. She had no idea what was wrong with her, and I knew I did not know why. This went on for months, the both of us trying to diagnose ourselves. When Vernetta was going through her physical trial, I had not yet been diagnosed.

On January 28, 1998, I was diagnosed with Hodgkin's disease. Vernetta was shocked, but I am sure she was not nearly as shocked as I was. She did everything in her power to encourage me. She continued to pray for me and try to bring me comfort while she was going through her own private hell. After I started my radiation treatments, Vernetta was compelled to go and see another doctor for the pain she was having in her lower back. I remember the phone call that literally broke my heart. I told you that she was a very calm person.

So, in her very serene and calm voice, she said to me, "T, now don't get upset about what I'm about to tell you."

At that time, I was feeling scared. Nothing could have prepared me for what she was about to tell me. "I have breast cancer."

"What?" I could not believe it. We both had cancer at the same time and did not know it, but little did either one of us know, Vernetta was the worse off.

Vernetta wanted to live. She was not ready to leave this life. She was a single woman who always desired to get married. She wanted to see her son become successful in the music industry. There were just too many things she desired to do.

We continued to pray, and when I could, I would go and visit her. She was slowly deteriorating and was soon in the hospice program. Vernetta never stopped believing God for her healing. The doctor wanted to remove the cancerous breast, but she did not want him to. She was determined to live and live completely, but she did not even have the support that I had. Yes, she had someone in the home with her. Her son and her daughter-in-law lived with her. They were present in the home, but they were not good caregivers.

There were many days that she did not eat until midday, and it was not because she did not want to eat. It was because her children were upstairs in bed until two o'clock in the day, but she never complained. She would just lie in her bed hoping that things would eventfully get better. There were times when I had to bring her food because the children had not fed her. It was heartbreaking to see her live like that. I wondered just how long she would be able to go through that.

She remained in good spirits all of the time, and she never complained. I would still call her to pray with her and encourage her. I do not know if she accepted that she was dying, but she never talked about it. Her courage was so profound, and her spirit was unmovable. I have never met anyone yet as remarkable or as humble as Vernetta. She definitely fought a good fight.

Vernetta succumbed to cancer on September 22, 1998. Although she left this physical realm, her spirit is still very prevalent to many people. She was a strong warrior in the spirit, and heaven is blessed for having her presence. When I saw her for the last time, she was gasping for each breath. Finally, her best friend told her to go on home.

"YOU CAN GO," she said.

Two hours after I left the hospital, Vernetta went home to be with the Lord. I thought that it would be befitting to devote an entire chapter to my friend because she taught me so much about love and friendship. Vernetta loved me unconditionally. Even at her lowest point, she could always manage to give me a smile. I LOVE YOU, VERNETTA, WITH ALL MY HEART!

The Inner Healing

$\mathbf{A}$s I reflect back on my illness, I am saddened because I know that my illness could have been avoided if I had not allowed myself to become entangled in practices that opened a gateway to this insidious disease. My lifestyle made me so vulnerable to this demon. I hope that what I am about to share with you will deliver you, if you are involved in these practices.

When I was a teenager, my mother introduced me to the world of witchcraft in the form of Ouija boards and readers (psychics). My mother was forever running to one to find out what they saw for her future. At that time in her life, she was a very unhappy woman who was looking for hope wherever she could find it. That same lust began to drive me as well. It became a ritual for me and other family members. I lived my life around what psychics foretold to me. As a result, I found it very difficult to desire and plan my own life or allow God to plan it. I felt that they were gifted, and what they said was the final word. This became a stronghold, and I knew I had to get away from that life, but not without paying the consequences first.

When I was in my late teens, around eighteen, I was introduced to a palm reader. She was an elderly white woman, and she read my palm and told me many things about my life. Some of them I do not care to mention, but one of the things she told me was that I was going to become very ill during mid-age, but I would come through it. I accepted what she said and went on with my life. Actually, I forgot about it. I was too busy trying to stop the other terrible things she had told me about from happening. I went on with my life, and shortly after that, my father was fighting cancer (lymphoma), and all I could think about was his suffering and the role I desired to play in relieving his pain.

Did You Know?

While modern technology, such as, 900 numbers and the Internet are partially responsible for fueling their recent popularity, psychics and mediums are not new. Psychic means, 'A person who is either born with or develops many gifts or talents in the area of ESP (extra sensory perception), clairvoyance, communication with the spirit world, abilities to read the human aura and uses these special skills as a healer or reader.'

The history of psychics can be traced back thousands of years ago to the seers, shamans, and soothsayers of ancient pagan religions and occult practices although it is relatively new in North America.

In the middle of the 19th century, the popularity of mesmerism and especially its alleged healing properties, along with the celebrated 'rappings' of the Fox sisters of Hydesville, New York, led directly to the sweeping acceptance of the

Spiritualist Movement of the later half of the 19th century.

However, the Bible does warn of demons, 'seducing spirits' and 'doctrines of devils' (I Timothy 4:1). Faith in psychics can be not only spiritually, but emotionally dangerous as well. Followers can become very dependent on their psychics for making even simple decisions. Psychics, in turn, can easily use their influence to control and take advantage of their clients

While I was in college, I went to visit him during the Christmas break one night. I could hear him moaning in agony because the pain was unbearable. My heart was grieved, and I would cry out to God and ask Him to allow me to bear my father's pain.

One evening, God spoke to me and said, "NO, because when it is time for you to bear your pain, no one will be able to relieve you of yours."

I did not understand at the time that God was foretelling my sickness. It was beyond my comprehension what God was preparing me for, but He soon revealed it to me on that fateful evening when He spoke to me, "This is a comma in your life, not a period."

As the night grew longer, the darkness in the room began to comfort me. God began to bring back to my remembrance what He told me many years ago when my father was ill. He revealed to me that I had opened up the door to this illness through witchcraft, and through harboring unforgiveness, bitterness, and strife in my heart. I also poisoned myself with the wrong types of foods because eating was the only satisfaction I had in life. Through all this, cancer entered into my body. He showed me that "you are what you eat" spiritually, emotionally, psychologically, and physically.

The cancer may have been diagnosed on January 28, 1998, but it took root that day I placed my palm in the hand of a witch. I accepted it. I did not fight back because I did not know that I had the authority to denounce that demon and send it back to where it came from. In addition, I was a very bitter woman because I felt betrayed and victimized all of the time. As a result, the self-hatred and hatred of others grew into cancer.

The silence of the room made God's voice appear more pronounced, and He continued to minister to me. He told me that He was going to do a work in me so that he could do a work through me. Then I could go and share His message of hope. He promised me that I was coming out of this situation, but first I had to go through it, and when I came through it, the greater work would be complete.

You see, He was not just concerned about my body. It was my damaged soul He wanted to heal and set free from the shackles that held me bound for so many years. He planned to equip me with the knowledge that would set others free. He told me that cancer is not just a tumor in the body, it is a deeply rooted foul seed that permeates our bodies in order to destroy our lives spiritually, emotionally, and psychologically. God is on a mission. He intends to use me and other survivors to annihilate this demonic force, bring restoration, and give hope to His people, not only from cancer, but also from every insidious disease.

Many of you may know that I am the author of the book *I Miss the Hugs but Not the Hurts*, which deals with coming out of toxic and codependent relationships. It talks about learning to love, respect, and accept yourself. I wrote this book after my cancer ordeal. I know it was that journey of being involved with the wrong men that placed me on the path of destruction. I know that my cancer came from being stressed out because I was in poor relationships with all those men in my past. I allowed myself to become smothered with that toxic spiritual, emotional, and psychological waste.

I did not like myself; therefore, I attracted the wrong men. I was a magnet for pain. Pain begets pain, and love begets love. I did not think I was worthy of having the best. Oh, I wanted to have someone worthwhile in my life, but I did not think someone like that would be attracted to me. I found myself settling for men who I knew I did not want as life companions. I just allowed myself to go through the motions. I stayed in la-la land in my imagination. I, somehow, convinced myself that we could make this work, but deep down inside, I knew I did not want them. I repeatedly asked myself, "WHY?" The answer was simply because I was emotionally, psychologically, and financially needy, and I wanted someone to fulfill those needs. Although my needs were many, I had hoped that the men I became involved with could help meet some of those needs.

It was not easy being a single mother with the responsibly of a house. Sometimes, I felt so overwhelmed, and to me the solution was having a man around to help with the load, but instead he just made things worse. I became so distraught and stressed out that it started to affect my health, unbeknownst to me. I went through being involved with the wrong men for about twenty-three years of my life, and it was taking its toll on me.

When I saw the palm reader, that was the beginning of my curse because she spoke it into existence. As you know, words have power, and it is very important that the words you speak about yourself and the words that others speak over you contain life, and not death or defeat.

Death and life are in the power of the tongue, and they that love it shall eat the fruit thereof (Proverbs 18: 21, KJV).

The men were just the fuel that ignited the flames. I realize now that I was a very bitter person, and pain was very prevalent in my life. I also held on to unforgiveness. It was inevitable that sickness would come into my body because like so many others, I did not really know how many of those events were damaging me.

When it comes to the laws of the land, ignorance of the law is no excuse, and the same is true for spiritual laws. Just because you do not know does not make you exempt from the consequences of defying that spiritual law. A lack of knowledge is the cause of many people meeting a premature death; even suffering through illness can be brought on by ignorance.

Now, I do not want anyone who has been ill to think that they were bad people and God punished them. I am merely saying be careful of your lifestyle because it can open up many doors that lead to destruction. You are what you eat, and your diet must consist of healthy and positive elements. It does not matter whether it is your natural diet or your spiritual one. What you allow yourself to ingest today will determine your fate tomorrow. You will reap what you sow. Unfortunately, I had to learn that lesson the hard way.

Through many trials and tribulations, some of which I could have possibly avoided; I learned a very valuable lesson. I learned that life is too long to be miserable, and when you are miserable, time seems to stand still. Self-love is the key to wellness, and love from others helps us to maintain that wellness. When that force is disturbed, then the body and the spirit faces destruction. Our bodies and spirits were created to work in sync. When God created man (Adam), He created us in His image. Death, sickness, and sorrow were never intended for man to experience.

My inner healing began when I realized that forgiveness was the beginning of healing. God instructed me to call everyone I could physically get a hold of and forgive them and let go of their offenses. I asked for forgiveness too, if I offended anyone. This was very challenging to me because I encountered many offenses during my illness, and I was afraid I would blow my healing. Please understand this fact, just because God told me He was going to heal me did not mean that it was going to come without paying a price. He told me I had to go through this ordeal because He wanted to do a work in me and through me. If I were not obedient to His command, I would have prolonged my sickness. It took nine months. Maybe, God wanted to do it in five or three months. I may never know, but I do know that many opportunities arose for me to be unforgiving and to harbor strife.

I had to believe God to heal me from cancer and from my wounded emotions and, on top of that, give me the desire to go on. There were many days that I wanted God to take me. The agony was killing me. No one knew how I felt. There were times when I did not want to talk to God. I refused to talk to Him. I was angry with Him because He allowed people to hurt me. My church hurt me. My family hurt me. I was all alone! The radiation and chemo was a breeze compared to the emotional anguish I experienced. I felt I was never going to get past that. I just knew it. That was how I felt for a long time, and it greatly affected how I went through my treatments too.

The treatments became more unbearable; I was sick all the time and very frustrated. Where was God now? It did not seem like I was getting any better. I was going through a great depression, and I wanted out of that situation. When I went to the clinic to get my chemo, I would get sick in the chair. On one occasion, I could not even finish the treatment. I knew my mother was struggling with having to see me like that, and I did not want to bother her with how miserable I was feeling. Her prayers became even more intensified. She had to pray for both of us because I stopped praying. All I could say to God was, "Have mercy, please!"

I would stare at the wall in a daze, not even knowing what I was thinking. Oftentimes my mind was blank as I still could not believe I was going through it. Wake me! This had to be a bad dream.

My only peace came in the stillness and silence of my dark room. I looked forward to the night and dreaded the day. I felt that my church misunderstood me and my family, the ones in Detroit, did not show enough concern. I was all messed up in the head. I did not know if it was the treatment or the devil working double overtime with me. I know, now, that it was the latter.

This feeling of hopelessness went on for months. Therefore, I guess God said, "Enough is enough." When I thought I had gone as low as I could go, He spoke to me in that still, quiet voice and asked me the question, "Do you want to die?"

I did not answer the question.

He asked me again. Then after the question, He made a statement. He said, "You may give up the ghost if you want to, but your spirit is not ready to leave you because it knows you have not finished your course. I have a great task for you to do for Me. I gave you My Word, that I am going to bring you through this, and you must go through this. I want to do a work in you, to do a work through you. My Word will come to pass that I spoke to you. So, come out of this slumber that you are in and LIVE! LIVE!"

God told me to live. God touched me, and it was at that moment that I realized no matter what I was going through, or how I felt or even how others were treating me, He had not abandoned me (Hebrews 13:5).

He was for me, and He was going to perform His work in this vessel no matter what (Philippians 1:6). It was at that moment I answered the question that He asked me. I answered, "No, I do not want to die, I want to live!" At that moment, my mission became even clearer to me, and my focus from that day forward was to get better so that God could use me. I was on a mission now, and I looked forward to embarking on it and completing it.

That ye put off concerning the former conversation the old man, which is corrupt according to the deceitful lusts; and be renewed in the spirit of your mind; and that ye put on the new man, which after God created in righteousness and true holiness (Ephesians 4:22-24, KJV).

"The cancer may have been diagnosed on January 28, 1998, but it took root that day I placed my palm in the hand of a witch."

The Victory

I am vibrant and beautiful. This is how I began to see myself. I started getting out more and enjoying the sunshine. My friend, Dee, would come over and take me for rides. She would encourage me to drive myself sometimes. My GMC Jimmy sat in the garage unless my son drove it. I had not driven since I drove myself to work the last day before going to emergency on January 28. It felt good to be in the driver's seat again. I was coming through my treatments just fine, and Dr. Fregene was very pleased with my progress. I was going on outings that were more social. People were beginning to see the glow and the calling on my life. I had an opportunity to go to Rev. Ron Coleman's church, God Land Unity, and he immediately began to exhort me. I believe it was my first time meeting

him, and he could see the Spirit of God all over me.
He told me that God was going to use me mightily,
and that I would have a healing ministry. Little did
he know that not only would it be a healing of the
body, but also a healing of the inner man. He
promised me that he would allow me to speak at
his church when I recovered from my illness. He
kept his word. I spoke at his church in July of 2001,
and I received two standing ovations. Guess what
my message was entitled? Yep, you guessed right,
*THIS IS A COMMA IN YOUR LIFE, NOT A
PERIOD.* There were other occasions also that
people noticed my new inner beauty. I had an
opportunity to work on the phone bank for Irma
Clark when she was running for state
representative (Michigan). Of course, she won, and
I attended her victory party. The Wayne County
clerk, Teola Hunter, approached me to tell me how
beautiful I was. She had never met me before. I
was so flattered that such a graceful woman
noticed me and took the time to tell me. We were in
the spring season, and I felt like I was going to
experience a new beginning. I was excited about
living again. I had already begun to map out what I
was going to do with my life once my treatments
were over. The spring season just seems to have

that affect on people, doesn't it?

I was invited to the graduation ceremony at Harris School to speak to the graduates. I took pictures with the staff. Although I was on a walker, they did not treat me any differently. I was beginning to see the hand of God in this whole ordeal. He had taken me through a spiritual metamorphosis. God had dealt with me on every level concerning my healing. He allowed me to see the source of my affliction. He showed me how I was to teach others about the gateway to destruction and how it can be avoided. Like Job, He did not afflict him, but He allowed it to happen. God did not afflict me, but because of the sin in my life, I was an open target for the enemy to overtake me. Anything contrary to the Word of God is dangerous. It does not matter whether or not you knew better. Ignorance of the law is not an excuse. There are spiritual principles put in place, and if we violate them, there are consequences that must be paid. Unfortunately, some have paid with their lives.

God began to show me how stress and bitterness upsets the harmony in our bodies. It is when this harmony is upset that the body begins to turn on itself. Our bodies were never designed to have diseases. In the Garden of Eden, Adam was a perfect specimen and so were his surroundings. Both were in tuned with God and His Word. When we allow negative forces in this world to overtake us, the enemy can hinder us with affliction. We must stay focused on the prize and not allow anything to deter us from achieving our dreams that God ordained for us to fulfill. I was not about to let go of the vision that He placed in me so many years ago. I was not going to give the grave another opportunity to put a gifted person six feet under. So many people have died prematurely because they did not deal with their issues. When I say died, I do not necessarily mean a physical death only. There are people walking around on this earth that are literally dead in their spirits. These are the drug addicts, the drunks, the prostitutes, the men in prison, and those who abuse his or her spouse.

There are children who would rather engage in gang wars rather than go to school. There are victims of HIV and AIDS because of sharing a dirty needle and/or having multiple sexual partners. Mothers who have several children out of wedlock and do not have a clue as to who the fathers are, but they choose to address their plight on the many talk shows. I can go on and on, but I believe you understand what I am saying. It is about choices! Choices that we make to live and fulfill our destiny.

On the other hand, we can walk around like the living dead. I decided to live and fulfill my destiny.

"We your servants will do as our LORD commands" (Numbers 32:25, NIV).

For God will bring every deed into judgment, including every hidden thing, whether it is good or evil (Ecclesiastes 12:14, NIV).

I knew I had to get busy living, so I started with the spiritual aspect of my life. I had a book that I read daily, written by Charles Capps on healing. It was a little pocket-size book with nothing but scriptures on healing in it. I read these scriptures when my energy permitted me. I knew that there would be days when I would be too weak. So, I decided to record the word on cassette. Those days when I was too weak to read, I played the recorder and allowed the words to minister to me. The goal was to listen to this recording daily when I was not able to read it. There were friends like the Bonners who gave me videotapes on healing and herbs to take. I was determined to get better quickly. I also read the Bible and prayed more. I began to visualize myself in complete, good health. There were times when God even used me to minister to others. There were several times when someone called to minister to me, and I ended up ministering to him or her. It was amazing to them that I was so unselfish during this time.

My sister in West Palm Beach played a major role in my recovery. She invested in my physical healing by purchasing me a juicer, the Champion, which I believe is the top of the line. She got in touch with her good friend, Anne Steele, who at the time was selling the juicer and Barley Green, which by the way is one of the best sources of beta-carotene you can take. The juicer was over $200, and my sister was not really in a position to buy it, but because of her love for me, she made the sacrifice. Anne came by to meet me and brought with her the juicer, a twenty-five-pound bag of carrots, some beets, and green apples to make me a juice tonic. When we met, we hit it off immediately. We fell in love with each other. Her spirit was so calm and gentle, and the serenity that she expelled was awesome. I was so comforted that she wanted to spend time with me and share in my recovery. I must say that I was very disappointed that Marlene did not come to visit me, but I suppose she made up for it by sending Anne.

I consumed this cancer-fighting tonic almost daily, and sometimes, two or three times a day. The

Barley Green was the most important ingredient though. This powder came from the baby barley plant. Then, brown rice and kelp was added to it to give it the healing components that worked so effectively. The Barley Green tasted like raw spinach, and I would mix it with the juice. The chemo was destroying all of the bad as well as the good cells in my body, so the juice and Barley Green helped build and create healthy cells in my body. Now, understand that some doctors do not agree with the holistic ways for healing. This is a decision that should be made with a lot of research.

My oncologist did not agree with me taking the tonic because I was taking a very strong chemo mixture. He did not think that the herb would be good with it. I felt like it could not hurt, and it did help boost my energy level. I am not a medical doctor, but if you are reading this book right now and you are a cancer patient or the family member or friend of one, I say to you that the object is to LIVE! Do not be afraid to ask questions about your treatments and explore new ones. There are a lot of progressive medicines and herbs out there that can help you defeat this killer. Be aggressive with this disease, and do not allow it to intimidate you. Love yourself in spite of your plight because it will be the love of yourself and others that will get you through your ordeal.

Plenty of fresh air and positive fellowship were the last ingredients to my victory. I began to install back into my days a social life. I surrounded myself with people who I enjoyed being around and who did not have a problem with my condition. This was excellent therapy for me. I wanted to live my life as normal as possible. It was important to me to feel normal. I went to the movies, out to dinner, to plays, and concerts. I recall even going to a spa to be pampered. Vaseline sponsored it. My mother and I went together.

It was important that self-examination took place with me. To my readers, this would be good for you too. Look at the areas of your life that need to be changed, and ask yourself if your healing is worth going through the deliverance God wants to subject you to. If you are ill, you cannot afford to allow bitterness and unforgiveness to brew. It will only cause your condition to worsen. I had to learn the hard way that God is not going to pacify you and condone your mess. The Word of God says that love covers a multitude of faults. That means that love is an excellent power and the ultimate medicine for any situation. Give yourself over to love and surround yourself with love. If there is someone in your life who is not giving you the love you need, then move on and find it from someone else. It is out there. Trust me, it is not worth settling for less than a perfect, unconditional love relationship with a person who respects you and nurtures you.

My victory came when I realized that God had an excellent way for me, and a great life was awaiting me. I had to let go of the dumb stuff and start living and taking control of my life. I let go of some people that were weighing me down spiritually and emotionally. I am still cleaning my spiritual and emotional house. I am happy about that too. God restored me and placed me in right standing with Him. This can happen for you because it is His perfect will. Be encouraged and allow God to put you in that perfect place so that you can experience your healing. Victory can be yours! I went through a horrific ordeal, and it has affected every area of my life. Please do not allow a doorway of destruction to entice you through poor choice making, lust, and poor self-esteem. This is my saga. God delivered me because of the calling that I have on my life. I am not trying to frighten you, but this may not be your story. This story is not only a story of hope, but it is also a warning. You are going to be held responsible for what you know, and if you are reading this book, then you will be without an excuse. Reaching your full potential is God's perfect will for your life. Anything short of that is a catastrophe. Do not get caught off guard. Be about the business of living, and make it your business to live!

This Is A Comma In Your Life, Not A Period

When people have cancer, life will change for them and the people who care about them. These changes in daily life can be difficult to handle. It is natural for a person with Hodgkin's to have many different and sometimes confusing emotions. I was often plagued with depression, and I was also angry and frightened about the future. Although I believed that I was going to come through that, I did not know how the rest of my life was going to be affected. Because I had extensive nerve damage to my lower spine, I did not know if I would be handicapped for the rest of my life. Presently, the tumors are gone, but it feels like I am carrying twenty-five pounds of dead weight around my waist. If you have ever worn a tight girdle around your waist, this is how it feels. Recovering from any type of cancer will probably prohibit you from having a very normal life again. I tell people that it is like being in a major car accident. You can fix up the outside of the vehicle, but the engine will never run the same. This is how cancer affects the body. I am cancer free, but I will continue to have a constant reminder of my ordeal. If that statement makes you question the validity of the miracle that God performed, remember it was more than just a physical healing. It was a time of restoration and redemption as well.

I had to get rid of the hindrances in my life, and I soon discovered who was for me and who was not for me. So many people stepped up to the plate to be a tremendous blessing to me, not only physically, but also spiritually. Sheryl Newberry was one of the soldiers God sent to me to help fight the battle. She and I spent a lot of time together, but during that time, she was very busy trying to get herself together. Being a former drug addict, she had many hurdles to overcome, and she was doing a fine job in overcoming them. She would call me from time to time just to keep in touch with me. Sheryl was crazy about me. I was her hero. I was there for her when she was at one of the lowest points in her life. I saw the goodness and the great potential in her when no one else did. You see, I met her when I was the manager of a homeless shelter, the Promise Land Community Shelter. She was one of the residents in the shelter. Although she was into that life, I could see that she was going to reach her destiny, and maybe I was to play a major role in the game plan. I had no doubt in my mind that she was going to get on her feet and discover just what God had in store for her. I was correct. Now, she is an ordained missionary on the battlefield for God, saving those who are as lost as she once was.

When Sheryl found out I was ill, immediately, she came to my aid. She came with the Bible in one hand and a bag of groceries in the other. She rolled up her sleeves and started to get busy doing whatever was needed—always praying and giving me encouraging words. She was not the least bit worried because she knew that this was a trial leading to a great work! I told her what God told me on the night of January 28 when I was sitting in the dark all alone in my living room: THIS IS A COMMA IN YOUR LIFE NOT A PERIOD!

She shouted with a loud, "Praise the Lord." It was almost as if she was glad I was going through so that God could do an excellent work in me through that ordeal.

There were days when I was so sick that I wanted to give up. She would not let me. She reminded me of the words He spoke to me, and she would hold my hand and pray with me. She would not leave my side until I fell asleep or she had to leave to go to work. I never felt so close to her as I felt at that time in my life. She became my rock and a strong anchor. To this day, she is my close friend, and she just beams at me every time she sees me. I do not think there is anyone in my life that admires me as much as she does. However, she is the one who should be admired because the power of God changed her life. She came a long way, and I am proud of her. She is my friend, and her kindness will always be remembered for helping me carry my cross when others stood by and were just spectators.

I mentioned earlier in this chapter how there were many people that came to the forefront to help me. I cannot devote a whole chapter or a paragraph giving all of them credit, but I must give credit to whom it's due. My friend Richard Jackson was a trooper. I cannot begin to say enough about how he blessed me during that ordeal. If it were not for Richard taking me to my chemo sessions, and seeing to it that there was food and money available for me, I do not know how my mom and I would have made it. Richard had that committed spirit that is a rare quality today. No one in my family was as concerned about me as he was. Richard is not a boyfriend or a relative. He was and still is a wonderful and committed friend.

When Richard found out I was ill, he was devastated. He did not know what to think. I believe that he was more concerned about whether or not I was going to get through this alive. I think that out of all of my friends, he took it the hardest.

You see, Richard has known me since I was in my early twenties, and he had become a very good friend of the family. Richard saw me go through some difficult times and watched me come out of them victoriously, and he admired my strength. He stuck by me through thick and thin, and he never gave up on me. When he found out that I was ill with cancer, I do not think he had the faith it took to believe I would pull through. Although I had slain some giants, he was not too sure I could slay this one. Please understand me, he was very positive and attentive, but I could see that he was often scared. I do not know what bothered him the most, the fact that I might die or that I might die and he would lose his friend. He could not see himself going through life without me being a part of it.

Richard did everything in his power to make me comfortable, and he even spoke to the oncologist to keep track of my progress. The doctor did not mind sharing it with him because he could see that Richard was very concerned. The last chemo treatment was the happiest day of Richard's life. He realized that I was going to make it. I do not remember if it rained or if the sun was out on that day, but for Richard, the sun was shining on the inside of his heart. It was as if he woke up from a nightmare. We celebrated by going out to dinner with my mother.

In September of 1998, Dr. Fregene released me to go back to work. I was cancer free. All the tests that I took during the month of August came back negative. I was able to resume my regular work schedule working from 9:00 a.m. to 9:00 p.m., Monday through Thursday and got off at 3:30 p.m. on Fridays. I continued this work schedule until the fall of 2002. I knew that I could not continue to work this schedule much longer because it was time to write this book, and I was going to need the time to write it. For years, I put off writing this book because of the pain that I felt. I knew in my spirit that the reader would only read and experience the pain I felt if I wrote it sooner. I had to allow my healing to take place before I could actually tell my story. I know that I am not a celebrity, and I am certainly not rich. I am just an ordinary person telling an extraordinary story about healing, deliverance, and restoration. I want to convey, as simply as I can, the goodness and mercy of a living God that thought enough of me to bring me through this. When I placed my hand in the hand of that palm reader, I had no idea that I was sealing my fate, but God intervened and changed the plan. What was intended for evil and destruction was turned around for good and victory. He took a situation intended for defeat and turned it into a ministry.

Many of you who are reading this book are ill or know someone who is ill. I am here to tell you that God is not a forsaker. He is a very present help in the time of a very present need (Psalms 46:1). Do not give up or get discouraged in your trial. Whether you are going through a bout with cancer or another disease, God is bigger than it is. The key to healing lies in the knowledge that forgiveness must take place first. Many illnesses come from unforgiveness and strife. If you are reading these words and you are ill or you know someone who is ill, let the healing begin from the heart. If someone has hurt you and you have not confronted it, now is the time. Remember, healing is for the one who feels victimized. Once you have confronted that issue, then and only then can the love of God come in and cleanse you. Love covers a multitude of faults. Guess what? That includes healing. If you ask anyone who is suffering with an illness, if there is someone that they have an ought against, if they are honest, they will answer yes. Sickness does not just come upon you overnight. It has been incubating for years. It has been lying dormant, just waiting for the right time to come forth. God revealed this to me.

I would like to make a few suggestions that will assist you in getting through an illness or preventing one:

1. I want to encourage you to take a moment to write down on a piece of paper all of the areas in your life that you have experienced pain. Once you can admit that you have been hurt and face it, the healing can begin.
2. Examine all of your relationships, and ask yourself who is just going along for the ride. Many of you have held on to people that you should have released a long time ago. They are toxic to you. Let them go. It does not matter if they are relatives, either. We

cannot help who our relatives are, but we can certainly select our friends.

3. Start taking control of your life. If it is not in your heart to do something, then do not do it. Oftentimes we find ourselves being men pleasers, and we end up being miserable in our lives.

4. If you are on a dead end job, RUN as fast as you can away from it. There is nothing more miserable than spending the first eight hours of your day doing something that you do not enjoy doing.

5. Find a hobby. All work and no play make Jane and James dull children.

6. Fall in love. Fall in love with yourself first, and then allow God to bring you that special someone. It is not good for man to be alone (Genesis 2:18). If you were to do research on the number of people who get ill, most of them are people who are alone or in relationships and are not happy in them.

7. Last but not least—change your diet. If you are ill, start eating more fruits and vegetables. Most of them are full of antioxidants (cancer fighters). And drink plenty of water. Eliminate sugars from your diet, such as, candy, cookies, cakes, etc. Get

familiar with a juicer, and begin to drink fresh juices, such as carrots, beets, and apples. I made a tonic from these ingredients, and it was great! I will be sharing the recipe with you later.

Let the healing begin! I have made seven suggestions that will aid you in the healing process or help prevent sickness from attacking you. I know that if you put these suggestions to practice in your life, you will see a tremendous change.

Your journey may not be like mine, but remember that it is a journey. I cannot tell you how long your journey will be, but I do believe that you will come through it. Your attitude will greatly determine just how much progress you make and what the prognosis will be. Even if you are not ill and your role is just to be an encouragement to someone who is ill, you play a very vital part to his or her recovery. If you took the time to read this book, then evidently, you want to know exactly what you need to do. I do not wish sickness on anyone, but if or when it comes, please do not allow yourself to think that you were a bad person and this is your punishment for all of your wrongdoings. No, do not think that way. Instead, think of it as an opportunity to allow God to work in and through you. Did you know that some of the most beautiful pottery that God created had to be placed in extreme heated conditions, but it came out to be a vessel of honor and He used it to be a blessing to many, many people? God is not finished with you yet. In fact, with some of you, He is just getting started. He is concerned more about the process than He is the beginning or the end. Allow Him to complete that perfect work in you (Philippians 1:6).

What may have been intended for evil can be turned around for His good. He has appointed the time and place for your perfection. Get out of the way, and allow Him to complete the work He has started. Always know this, that God knows the end of the thing. When it looks bleak and you feel that you cannot make it another step, remember the comforting words He spoke to me on that dark wintry evening, "THIS IS A COMMA IN YOUR LIFE, NOT A PERIOD!" Let these words bring healing to your heart and to your situation. He is faithful to finish the work He has begun in you. Get excited, and let the blessings of God overtake you.

But as for you, you meant evil against me; but God meant it for good, in order to bring it about as it is this day to save many people alive. Now therefore, do not be afraid; I will provide for you and your little ones. And he comforted them and spoke kindly to them (Genesis 50:20-21, NIV).

And behold a woman, which was diseased with an issue of blood twelve years, came behind him and touched the hem of his garment. For she said within herself, if I may touch his garment, I shall be whole. But Jesus turned him about, and when he saw her, he said, "Daughter, be of good comfort; thy faith hath made thee whole" (Matthew 9:20-22, KJV).

Conclusion: Finishing Strong

Life will bring challenges that we are not always prepared for, and they may even take us to a place where we feel disconnected and alone. I shared my experience with you, and today, I am not the person that I was nine years ago. Today, I walk in purpose and victory. I actually look forward to life and fulfilling my destiny. I want you to do the same.

I want to encourage you to look up and look forward to a brighter today by making good choices. Let go of the past and surround yourself with people who love you and have your best interest at heart, and finally, and this is most paramount— FORGIVE.

Many of the snares we face are due to unresolved issues from our past, and unknowingly, we open up doors for many obstacles we encounter in life. But the message that God wants us to receive is this: Many are the afflictions we will face in our lifetime, but God is willing and able to deliver us from them all (Psalms 34:19). This is not an empty promise, it is a fact. God will not forsake you..

Do not allow yourself to think that God is punishing you if you are experiencing horrific challenges in your life. Yes, He is a God of wrath, but more so, He is a loving and faithful father who chastises us for perfection. God is concerned about the process, and He is well aware of the outcome. Therefore, think of your challenges as an opportunity to allow God to create a vessel of honor and one that can be used for purpose (2 Timothy 2:21). He has made a great investment in you, and He protects His investment and guards it.

Whatever your challenges are, you can go through it. Whether it is dealing with sickness, financial matters, death of a loved one, or the breakdown of a long-term relationship, whatever it may be, you can have the victory and finish strong.

I recall, after I thought my ordeal was over and I had gone back to working my grueling nine to nine schedule, I was concerned about my face and my neck. They both were swollen, and I made an appointment to see Dr. Fregene. It was about two months after I returned to work. I went to St. John Riverview Hospital for my visit because he also had an office there. He examined me and ran some tests; then he released me to go home. I was walking down the hallway getting ready to exit the hospital when a nurse hurried to stop me. She then told me that Dr. Fregene needed to see me again immediately.

"Now what?" I asked myself. I was on my way back to work because I had scheduled to see him on my lunch break, and my supervisor knew I was going to be a little late, and she had no problem with that. I turned around and walked back to Dr. Fregene's office, and he informed me that I was not going back to work, but I would be spending the night, and I was going to have surgery. What! I could not believe it. The swelling in my face and neck was due to the Metaport being in too long, and my main artery, the aorta, was being affected by it. I am not a doctor, so in laymen's terms, I was facing another near-death experience.

After that finding and a few other close calls, and after my initial ordeal with cancer, I began to see what God was really doing. He was letting me know He was still perfecting me and looking out for my best interest. I was still in recovery, and my total healing was a process, but I could still expect a full restoration in my health and every other area in my life.

Very shortly after the cancer ordeal, I began to reflect, and I remembered the question God asked me on that very dismal, lonely, and one of the worse evenings of my life, "Do you want to die?" I remember where I was spiritually and how I felt at that precise moment, very hopeless, helpless, and very much alone. I remember thinking about the hurts, the lack in my life, and my body poisoned with toxic tumors. At that time, the fight appeared to be in favor of my enemy. Soon after the question was answered and I told Him I wanted to live, but not only did I want to live, I wanted to live—*well.* It dawned on me that in order to do that I had to change. Cancer was introduced into my body because I opened the gateway for the intrusion.

God gave me a mandate. Teach others what I truly learned from this experience. In the preceding chapter I listed seven things to do to avoid sickness, but I am going to give you four keys or golden nuggets that will assist you in obtaining victory for no matter what you are going through in your life. If you keep them in mind and put them to practice, you will learn how to come out, avoid, and stay out of life's atrocities.

1. GET OUT OF TOXIC RELATIONSHIPS. Get out of toxic relationships, and stay out of them. One of the primary reasons for my constant unhappy state of mind was due to me selecting the wrong men. I had my own baggage; I did not need their baggage too. Oftentimes, we select the wrong people because we do not know our self-worth, and we are very needy, emotionally and psychologically. We become a magnet attracting the wrong people, both romantically and platonically. This even applies to your family and business relationships. Any relationship that is not contributing positively to your life, let it go. The following points will encourage you to get out of toxic relationships:

- Trust that you desire better in your relationships, and expect it.
- Work on your issues and make sure you are not the hindrance.
- Surround yourself with people who are in healthy, nurturing relationships.
- Respect yourself—respect is not based on what is showing on the outside, but by what is on the inside that is reflected on the

outside.
- Preparation is not lost time. Use your "alone time" to work on some of your short -term and long-term goals. Go inside of yourself to explore the untapped gifts and talents you possess.

2. FORGIVE AND LET GO OF THE PAST. Anger and grief are a part of life, but when you are harboring unforgiveness and you let bitterness seep in, these emotions began to consume you, they begin to poison every area of your life. Unforgiveness is cancerous and opens the doors to other insidious diseases. Unforgiveness keeps you locked in the past and stifles your future. The following are suggestions to overcome unforgiveness and letting go of the past:

- Admit you are hurting and/or angry and you are having difficulty forgiving. Remember, forgiveness does not happen overnight, depending on how deeply rooted the pain is; it can be a long process.
- Separate yourself, if possible, from the individual you are angry with so that God can begin to deal with your heart.

- Seek counsel—go to a professional counselor, your local clergy, or a friend you can trust to talk out your anger and hurt. A sounding board is good therapy.
- Forgiveness is for you as well as the other person who offended or hurt you. But by you forgiving, the healing process begins.
- Daily affirm that you are letting it go and get busy living.

3. LOVE YOURSELF—ACCEPT WHO YOU ARE BEFORE YOU BECOME WHAT YOU CAN BE. Sometimes the hardest person to love is ourselves, and we often try to compensate for the self-dislike through our jobs or careers. Some even go as far as surgically altering their bodies. The person in the mirror is not always the real you, but the person we see in the mirror is a direct result of the real person on the inside. This is the area we should work on first, and the great transformation will be seen on the outside. The following suggestions will help you love and accept yourself:

- Begin to work on improving your character, personality, and physical flaws.

- Identify your best qualities and flaunt them.
- Affirm that you are God's best creation.
- Make it your business to look your best daily.
- Change your eating habits because your diet also affects your emotional, physical, and spiritual well-being.
- Eliminate stress in your life. It is one of the major factors for physical illness and poor life choices. FYI, when you are under stress, your immune system is ineffective for up to six hours, making you susceptible to sickness and disease.

4. MAKE THE RIGHT CHOICES. Making the right choices is probably the most difficult thing to do sometimes especially when we do not know what to do in a particular situation. Many of my poor choices were done because of a lack of knowledge and not having the right people around me to seek advice from or not utilizing other resources to get the information. I have always told my son, "If you do not know what to do in a certain situation, do nothing. Stand still. Then seek out counsel from reliable sources."

The following points will help you make better choices:

- Seek out Godly counsel by two or three people, preferably those who are knowledgeable about the subject matter.
- Make informed decisions—do your research.
- Weigh out the pros and cons before making a commitment to any major life choices.
- Consider the timing before you make a move.
- Consider the cost. Ask yourself, am I mentally, emotionally, and financially up to the challenge?

I believe very strongly that if you put these golden nuggets to practice, you will be well on your way to victory in every area of your life. God has nothing but good intentions toward you, and He has already mapped out your course, even the diversions. I have always said that God is not caught off guard, and He knows the end of the thing. Life may have a few battles, but rest assure that you will win the war. The battle is not given to the swift or the strong, but to whoever endures to the end. Constantly remind yourself that hardships and mishaps often build character and prepare us for a greater cause. God will take your misery and turn it into your ministry and give you the calling to encourage others to finish strong on their journey to emotional, physical, and spiritual healing.

> *"For I know the plans I have for you,"*
> *declares the Lord, "plans to prosper*
> *you and not to harm you, plans to*
> *give you hope and a future."*
>   (Jeremiah 29:11, NIV)

Super Antioxidant Tonic

Remember this tonic is not a cure for cancer, but it is a great source of antioxidants. If taken on a regular basis along with much faith and prayer, you can begin to see a difference in your health. Many doctors are not into natural healing and may discourage eating like this. I am not telling anyone not to take their medication or their treatments.

Remember, your objective is to live! One of the primary reasons that many people die is because they cannot eat. They lose their appetite. When this happens, taking this tonic can really create a tremendous source of nutrients for the body. Again, I am not a doctor. I am only telling you what worked for me. I also had extensive chemotherapy and radiation therapy. Prayer and being around positive people were also key factors that aided me during this ordeal.

TONIC RECIPE

25 lb bag of carrots
Raw beets
Green apples—granny apples
Fresh spinach (optional)
Barley green by AIM (This can only be purchased by a distributor or the manufacturer. 1-800-456-2462).

Note: If you do not have a juicer, this would be an excellent time to invest in one. I would recommend the Champion. Retails for about $250.

Wash and brush vegetables. Make sure that you peel the raw beets. You do not need to peel the apples or scrape the carrots. The vegetable brush will be sufficient for the carrots. You will use about three to four large carrots for juicing (single serving), double if preparing for more than one person. Juicing does not have to be in any particular order. Cut up one raw beet in sections so that it will fit into the mouth of the juicer. Cut green apple into four to six sections so it will also fit into the mouth of the juicer. You may add fresh spinach—not frozen or canned. When you have completed juicing, add one tablespoon of Bar Green to the juice, and mix well. You may want to purchase a miniature blender. Very important! Juice loses its potency after a few hours. When you juice, you should be ready to drink it immediately. Drink tonic at least twice a day. The tonic should be taken along with other well-balanced meals. If you can avoid red meat and sugar, please do so.

If you are wondering if this tonic is only for cancer patients, the answer is NO. Taking this tonic on a regular basis will serve as an excellent preventative source. This tonic will cleanse your system and give you a burst of energy. It helps maintain healthy cells. Here's to your health!

WHAT CANCER CANNOT DO

Cancer is so limited—
It cannot cripple love,
It cannot shatter hope,
It cannot corrode faith,
It cannot eat away peace,
It cannot destroy confidence,
It cannot kill friendship,
It cannot shut out memories
It cannot silence courage,
It cannot invade the soul,
It cannot reduce eternal life,
It cannot quench the Spirit,
It cannot lessen the power of the
Resurrection.

By the late Lucille Moore, deceased March 30, 1990

THIS IS A COMMA IN YOUR LIFE, NOT A PERIOD

This is a comma in your life, not a period, This is but a moment in time, but it is not the end. The odds may appear to be against you and the journey long and dry.
The mountain is hard to climb, but remember, it will take your footsteps to the sky.

In your search for peace, you will find it.
In your search for strength, you will embrace it.
In your search for faith, you will stretch it to its greatest length and call upon wisdom to guide you and counsel you in your most difficult quest.

Victory awaits you at the end of the road, and men and heaven's angels will applaud your courageous efforts to succeed.
You carried your cross, you endured the pain, and now the earth whispers your name.
You will be known for your courage and endurance, and credited for carrying a flame of faith.

You faced your trials head-on, and you overcame your enemy of fear.
They are no longer your companions because you

battled them with great tenacity.

You made up your mind to live, and you made up your mind to strive, and fate has turned the tables of life, and now in your future you will thrive.
You have learned a valuable lesson, and with wisdom, you will keep it near. For whenever life's challenges come and try to overtake you, just remember these words . . .

This is a comma in your life, not a period.
This is but a moment in time, but it is not the end
This is a comma in your life, not a period.

Written by

Dr. Tunishai Anne Ford

Book Highlights
From
This Is A Comma In Your Life, Not A Period

THE MOMENT OF TRUTH

"I knew that I was about to go through the most horrific experience of my life, but I knew God would be with me."

THE PROGNOSIS AND TREATMENT

"I was about to begin my journey to Gethsemane, and I knew my cross was going to be heavy, but little did I know God was going to send some Simons."

"Do not think because God gives you a word that faith does not have to be applied to it. Trust me, if I had not stood in faith, I would have died. We can abort the Word with our actions and our words."

"I knew I had to begin preparing myself for the journey of a lifetime. Therefore, I asked God to lead the way."

"This was a journey that no one or nothing could have prepared me for, but as my father would always say, 'I was going to come out, smelling like a rose.'"

RUDE AWAKENING

"Remember, love and sacrifice may not always afford us the opportunity to have it take place at an ideal time when we want to help or spend our money. When we truly walk in love, convenience will not be an issue in our work of faith."

"God did not make man to be a Lone Ranger. He did not place us each on a deserted island to be alone, but instead, He made us sociable beings to be concerned and caring toward one another."

"You have to ask yourself how far you want to go with your involvement with someone who is ill because you may never know when an illness will come upon you. You may need someone to 'GO ALL THE WAY!'"

"The principle is that if you sow good seed, it will surely come back to you. Likewise, the same is true if you do not sow seed at all, then you have nothing coming back."

"I learned firsthand that God will move with or without man."

"It is only by the Spirit of God that a person can be unselfish and giving during times of need."

"Ask what is needed. It might just be a friendly conversation or a nice long drive just to feel the wind on his or her face."

"Remember, when you least expect tragedy or hardship to come, it will. Ask yourself if you were there for someone during his or her time of need. If you were, rest assure that someone will be there for you."

"Prayer is not always enough. We should know that faith requires us doing if we have the ability to do for our brothers and sisters."

GOD HEARS A MOTHER'S PRAYER

"Moreover, it was during this time that I learned that my mother was truly a spiritual woman and had a direct pipeline with God."

"She was a woman who could not tell you where a scripture was found, and probably if she could, she would misquote it, but she believed that God could do anything but fail. She prayed a fervent prayer from her heart and was consistent."

"I did pray daily, but I believe that my mother's prayers touched and moved God."

"I strongly believe; in fact, I know that it was all because of the prayers of my mother and others that caused intervention to take place."

"When a mother cried out to Him for her child, He heard it, and the blessings that availed were unlimited."

"When I look in the mirror, I see her dreams in my eyes, and my thoughts are forever striving to fulfill her vision for me."

AN ANGEL NAMED TEE

"God sent someone who was kind and under standing to help me."

"It is not every day that you meet some one who is willing to show kindness without getting something in return or allowing himself or herself to get so involved with someone, even when it is not a close friend or relative."

"Because we live in a very apathetic world, it matters when someone goes out of his or her way to care."

"Do not force what is not meant to be. People are sent into our lives for different reasons. Some will pass through it, and others will stay longer. Be grateful that essence was given to you."

VERNETTA'S SONG

"Vernetta was like a beautiful flower in the midst

of cactus plants because she was so radiant, and nothing ever seemed to disturb her peace."

"Her courage was so profound, and her spirit was unmovable. I have never met anyone yet as remarkable or as humble as Vernetta. She definitely fought a good fight."

"She was a strong warrior in the spirit, and heaven is blessed for having her presence."

INNER HEALING

"When it comes to the laws of the land, ignorance of the law is no excuse, and the same is true for spiritual laws."

"Just because you do not know does not make you exempt from the consequences of defying that spiritual law."

"A lack of knowledge is the cause of many people meeting a premature death; even suffering through illness can be brought on by ignorance."

"Now, I do not want anyone who has been ill to think that they were bad people and God punished them. I am merely saying be careful of your lifestyle because it can open up many doors that lead to destruction."

"You are what you eat, and your diet must consist of healthy and positive elements. It does not matter whether it is your natural diet or your spiritual one. What you allow yourself to ingest today will determine your fate tomorrow."

"I learned that life is too long to be miserable, and when you are miserable, time seems to stand still."

"Self-love is the key to wellness, and love from others helps us to maintain that wellness."

"When that force is disturbed, then the body and the spirit faces destruction."

"Our bodies and spirits were created to work in sync. When God created man (Adam), He created us in His image. Death, sickness, and sorrow were never intended for man to experience."

"My inner healing began when I realized that forgiveness was the beginning of healing."

"Please understand this fact, just because God told me He was going to heal me did not mean that it was going to come without paying a price. He told me I had to go through this ordeal because He wanted to do a work in me and through me."

THE VICTORY

"God began to show me how stress and bitterness upsets the harmony in our bodies. It is when this harmony is upset that the body begins to turn on itself. Our bodies were never designed to have diseases."

"When we allow negative forces in this world to overtake us, the enemy can hinder us with affliction."

"We must stay focused on the prize and not allow anything to deter us from achieving our dreams that God ordained for us to fulfill."

"So many people have died prematurely because they did not deal with their issues."

"It was important that self-examination took place with me. To my readers, this would be good for you too. Look at the areas of your life that need to be changed, and ask yourself if your healing is worth going through the deliverance God wants to subject you to."

"The Word of God says that love covers a multitude of faults That means that love is an excellent power and the ultimate medicine for any situation."

"God restored me and placed me in right standing with Him. This can happen for you because it is His perfect will."

"Be encouraged and allow God to put you in that perfect place so that you can experience your healing. Victory can be yours!"

"Reaching your full potential is God's perfect will for your life. Anything short of that is a catastrophe."

"Do not get caught off guard. Be about the business of living, and make it your business to live!"

This Is A Comma In Your Life, Not A Period!

"I am here to tell you that God will not forsake you. He is a very present help in the time of a very present need (Psalms 46:1)."

"Whether you are going through a bout with cancer or another disease, God is bigger than it is."

"The key to healing lies in the knowledge that forgiveness must take place first. Many illnesses come from unforgiveness and strife."

"Remember, healing is for the one who feels victimized. Once you have confronted that issue, then and only then can the love of God come in and cleanse you. Love covers a multitude of faults."

"I cannot tell you how long your journey will be, but I do believe that you will come through it."

"Did you know that some of the most beautiful pottery that God created had to be placed in extreme heated conditions, but it came out to be a vessel of honor, and He used it to be a blessing to many, many people? God is not finished with you yet."

"What may have been intended for evil can be turned around for His good. He has appointed the time and place for your perfection."

"Always know this, that God knows the end of the thing."

TO CONTACT Dr. Tunishai Ford
For speaking engagements, workshops
Or to purchase additional copies of
Her book and other products,
email her at *Tunishai@sbcglobal.net*
or visit her website at *www.drtford.com.*